HEALTH MANPOWER PLANNING IN TURKEY

THE JOHNS HOPKINS MONOGRAPHS IN INTERNATIONAL HEALTH

HEALTH MANPOWER IN A DEVELOPING ECONOMY: TAIWAN, A CASE STUDY IN PLANNING. 1967.
by Timothy D. Baker and Mark Perlman

THE HEALTH CENTER DOCTOR IN INDIA. 1967.
by Harbans Takulia, Carl E. Taylor, Prakash Sangal, and Joseph D. Alter

HEALTH AND DISEASE IN FOUR PERUVIAN VILLAGES: CONTRASTS IN EPIDEMIOLOGY. 1968.
by Alfred A. Buck, Thomas T. Sasaki, and Robert I. Anderson

HEALTH MANPOWER PLANNING IN TURKEY

An International Research Case Study

by Carl E. Taylor, Rahmi Dirican, and Kurt W. Deuschle

The Johns Hopkins Press, Baltimore, Maryland

PREFACE

No other component of health services is as important as health manpower. In fact, the quality and organization of everything else from facilities to administrative structure, and especially public demand and response, will be determined largely by the capability and interests of the health personnel. The health sector is one of the most labor-intensive areas of development activity. As technology advances so must the preparation and ability of the human resources required to protect the health of modern man.

Health planners face a constant dilemma in trying to define the quantitative-qualitative balance of personnel appropriate for particular times and places. The recurring issue is whether to use limited resources for a few top-level professionals or to produce larger numbers of technical auxiliaries who can concentrate on simple approaches to mass problems.

The usual decision is to start both at the top and bottom in the hope of developing a symmetrical health manpower pyramid. Instead, most developing countries now have a manpower hourglass as a result of the following unplanned sequence. Any country or society has some continuation of the system of indigenous curative practice which traditionally provided mass medical care. With the introduction of scientific medicine, the urban elite tends to monopolize the relatively limited resources for sophisticated medical care. Charity facilities are quickly overwhelmed.

The first step in a country's health manpower development is usually taken at the top. Medicine is a prestigious career goal for highly educated upper-class youth. Having a medical school becomes an important status symbol for the country, then for every major city. A top-heavy manpower bulge of doctors in urban and hospital practice develops even where health services are nationalized.

Spontaneous political pressures, however, require some attention to the simple and obvious health needs of the general population. Rational considerations lead to concentration on mass preventive measures such as vaccination and DDT spraying because of the evident cost-benefit returns. But the villager is more interested in his immediate pains, sores, and fevers and in the running eyes, noses, and bowels of his children. The limited government and charity medical service have shown him that for certain conditions apparently magical cures can be obtained by injections and surgery. Confidence in indigenous practitioners starts to break down. If the government does not provide mass medical services, many entrepreneurs will move into this obvious demand vacuum. The fact that rural people have little available money merely means that the mass need will be met by low-level, local personnel and within the village economy.

Turkey provides a typical illustration of the manpower sequence that has been described. The manpower hourglass has some 10,000 doctors in its upper segment. Middle-level manpower is squeezed into a narrow belt with less than 2,000 diploma nurses and related paramedical categories and even fewer technical assistants of other categories. The great bulge in the lower segment of the manpower hourglass includes over 30,000 needlemen, who are often former army "medics" practicing independently in their home villages, and 40,000 untrained indigeneous midwives.

Manpower planning is an attempt to rationalize the present spontaneous and often cyclic trends. The social and economic forces of open market mechanisms have controlled private health services but with frequent lags and a tendency to overcompensation. Delays in the production of high-priority manpower categories and major gaps in services with gross social inequities to special groups have become particularly common, especially under the stresses of rapid economic growth in a developing country. Health manpower planning introduces scientific analysis which permits prediction of shortages, systematic attention to high-priority activities, and deliberate equalization of services.

Among the specific items that attracted our attention in Turkey were the sociological aspects of manpower planning such as the prejudice against nursing for middle- and upper-class girls and the generally prevalent negative attitudes toward rural practice among physicians. The most critical issues for government administrative policy relate to the feasibility of using greater numbers of auxiliary health personnel and improved mechanisms for providing supervision in the new plan for nationalized health services.

The Turkish Health Manpower Study was started in July, 1963, as a co-operative project between the Ankara School of Public Health under the Ministry of Health of Turkey and the Division of International Health of the School of Hygiene and Public Health of The Johns Hopkins University. Dr. Carl E. Taylor, director; Dr. Kurt Deuschle, field director; and Miss Alice Forman, public health nurse and research associate formed the United States team. Dr. Necat Erder was appointed project co-ordinator and Dr. Rahmi Dirican, chief investigator, under the general direction of Dr. Nusret Fisek, Undersecretary of the Ministry of Health. Dr. Dirican was later appointed project co-ordinator.

There were two clearly defined sets of objectives as this research project was organized.

1. Turkish planners and educators were interested in practical questions of how the health needs of Turkey could best be met. The first five-year plan, prepared in 1963, introduced the concept of national planning and demonstrated the need for new methodology and competence in health planning. There was much discussion of the need for radically altering medical and nursing education. This study, therefore, attempted to:

(a) define the present numbers and classifications of health personnel;

(b) identify imbalances in geographical, rural-urban, or social distributions of personnel providing health services;

(c) study utilization patterns of health services and determine present demand for health services in order to identify areas of unmet demand and to project these over a fifteen-year period;

(d) analyze economic factors controlling the potential expansion of health services and the equitable compensation of each category of health manpower;

(e) study educational trends and possibilities for modifying the output and preparation of each category of personnel to fit desired utilization patterns;

(f) explore various possibilities of improving the quality and efficiency of health services within present resources;

(g) evaluate the pilot projects of the national health services and make suggestions for improving the national plan.

2. The Johns Hopkins Division of International Health undertook this study with the financial support of the U.S. Agency for International Development, primarily to improve the methodology of health manpower research. Studies were undertaken simultaneously in Turkey, Taiwan, Peru, and Nigeria. At the time, research methodology was still in a rudimentary stage of development. Studies in more developed countries had concentrated mostly on the supply side of the equation. Demand standards were

arbitrarily based on personnel to population ratios which had evolved spontaneously. The shortages which are almost uniformly reported result partly at least from the standards used, since both the public and professionals are seldom satisfied with health services. But to measure and project both effective demand and supply of health manpower requires new technical sophistication and much imagination in methodological innovation.

During this research a series of specific studies were conducted to gather data in the following problem areas:

(a) tracing and identifying the supply of professionals and auxiliaries with particular attention to those categories on whom official records showed no information since their original registration—doctors' census, nurses' census, indigenous health workers' survey from village headmen;

(b) defining major difficulties of medical practice and doctor utilization—doctors' detailed questionnaire, private practitioners' reports on their patients;

(c) identifying the major professional problems of nurses—nurses' detailed questionnaire;

(d) estimating cost of medical services and doctors' income—doctors' census, doctors' detailed questionnaire, economic analysis of selected institutions;

(e) determining problems of rural health services—doctors' attitudes toward rural service, evaluation of nationalization of health services;

(f) evaluating medical education—survey of medical schools, cost of medical education;

(g) estimating unmet demand for health services—doctors' detailed questionnaire, private practitioners' reports on their patients, analysis of costs of health services and selected institutions.

A project of this magnitude is uniquely a team effort. A number of persons contributed from their official positions in the Turkish government, AID, educational institutions, and voluntary agencies. Many more provided active support in their private capacities and this includes, of course, the many health professionals of Turkey who were the primary objects of study. The final meetings in Ankara for evaluation and implementation proved important largely because of the contributions of cabinet ministers, directors of the various divisions of the Ministry of Health and the State Planning Organization, professors from most of the medical schools and other educational institutions, and representatives of the different occupational groups.

In addition to those already mentioned the Turkish field team included: Ustun Kusefoglu, Ayten Geray, Gulseren Gunce, Sukriye Karaosmanoglu, Hayrettin Kurama, Kenan Somer, Ahmet Tugac, Aysel Alpay, Ismail Issever, Ahmet Avcibasi, Mehmet Ogec, Zekeriya Avare, Yilmaz Doganlar, Avni Gundogdu, Sukru Ogec, and Pervin Sanci,

Also, many members of the faculty of the Ankara School of Public Health actively participated in the data gathering. We appreciated being given the opportunity to add questions to the two national surveys conducted by the State Institute of Statistics, and the Test Bureau of the Ministry of Education and the Population Council.

In the statistical analysis we relied mainly on the advice of Dr. William Reinke and Dr. Keith Watson. Dr. Mark Perlman and Mr. James Lancaster assisted with portions of Chapter 3. Much of the detailed work of preparing the manuscript was capably handled by Mrs. Sue Flanigan, editorial assistant of the Department of International Health. The main burden of typing the many drafts was cheerfully carried by Miss Carol Buckley with the assistance of Mrs. Martha List.

HEALTH MANPOWER PLANNING IN TURKEY

1

TURKEY: A COUNTRY IN TRANSITION

From early Hittite times through the Greek, Persian, Roman, and Byzantine periods Turkey has been a meeting place of the world's leading civilizations. In the tenth century, Central Asian nomads, under a leader named Seljuk, migrated to Anatolia and eventually conquered the land. Two centuries later their power was shattered by the Mongol invasion. As the Mongols withdrew, another nomad tribe, the Ottoman Turks, gained control. Ottoman expansion into Europe was facilitated by the weakness of the Byzantine Empire. Ultimately the Ottomans controlled Asia Minor, much of the Arabian peninsula, North Africa, the islands of the eastern Mediterranean, the Balkans, the Caucasus, and Crimea. A slow decline began late in the seventeenth century with final disintegration of the empire after World War I.

In 1919, with the Greeks invading western Anatolia, Mustafa Kemal, later Kemal Ataturk, led the fight for independence. On October 29, 1923, Turkey was declared a republic and the first democratic government was established under Ataturk. Dramatic steps were taken to achieve rapid Westernization. The caliphate was abolished and the caliph banished. Islamic law was replaced by a secular legal system based on Swiss and Italian law. A modified Roman alphabet supplanted the Arabic script in 1927. Women were granted the right to vote in 1934. A forced industrialization plan was launched but little was done to improve the primitive agricultural conditions, except for a widespread effort in rural education.

In spite of her nonparticipation in World War II, the cost of military defense has imposed a heavy burden on Turkey's economy. Turkey still allocates a larger percentage of her budget for military defense than any other country in the Western Alliance.

Economic development was somewhat accelerated after 1949 by foreign assistance, mechanization of agriculture, and an artificial economic expansion promoted by abundant imports. This advance was, however, largely neutralized by the population increase of 3 percent annually. During the twelve-year interval between 1948 and 1960, the rate of population increase was 66 percent of the rate of increase in the national industrial product.[1] Although both national income and agricultural output had more than doubled, per capita ratios showed only a 25 percent increase.

A military coup in May, 1960, led to a new constitution and particular emphasis on national planning. The first Five-Year Plan started in 1963 with the long-term target of a 7 percent annual growth rate in the gross national product (GNP) over a fifteen-year period. According to all recent national indices, Turkey is still a "developing country." The present 5.3 percent (1965 GNP growth) rate of growth[2] of the Turkish economy is lower than that of most European countries. The per capita GNP in 1961 was $199, as compared to $355 in Greece, $601 in Italy, $1,178 in France, and $2,717 in the U.S. (all 1959 figures).

SYSTEM OF GENERAL EDUCATION

The Educational Sequence

The total educational system of Turkey provides the educated manpower pool from which physicians and other health personnel are to be drawn. The serious problems which permeate general education provide a perspective for understanding the special problems of medical schools and other schools for health personnel.

Turkish education is almost entirely publicly supported, with private education accounting for only 0.3 percent of all enrollment in primary and secondary schools. Since 1923 public education has been free at all levels. All schools are controlled by the Ministry of Education. The structure of the educational system with approximate numbers of students is summarized in Table 1-1.

Although it is compulsory for all children between seven and fourteen to attend five years of primary school, only 70 percent of primary-school-age children were enrolled in the 1961/62 academic year. Secondary schools are of two types—those for general education and those for vocational and technical education (Table 1-1). In 1961/62, 25 percent of secondary-school-age children were in general education (middle school and lycee) and 7 percent were in technical and vocational schools (middle and high). A student who passes his primary-school leaving examination may choose to continue his studies in either a middle school or in one of the vocational and technical schools. Selection among the several avenues of education after primary school is usually based on family pressure, proximity of the school, and intensity of personal interest.

TABLE 1–1. THE EDUCATIONAL SYSTEM OF TURKEY, WITH NUMBER OF
STUDENTS AND TEACHERS AT EACH LEVEL (1961)

Type of school	School-age population ('000's)	Total no. of students ('000's)	Children attending school as % of school-age population	No. of teachers ('000's)	Student/ teacher ratio
Primary	4,613.0	3,160.0	70	67.9	46
Middle	1,786.0	333.0	19	5.2	64
Middle tech. & vocational		68.4	4	8.0	14
Lycee	1,505.0	86.0	6	2.5	34
High tech. & vocational		46.5	3	8.0	14
Higher university	1,816.0	51.0	3	2.8	19
Advanced technical & vocational		10.0	1	1.3	8

Source: First Five-Year Development Plan (State Planning Organization, Ankara) Table 357, p. 402.

Secondary education starts with three years of middle school, either general or vocational. The second or lycee stage also lasts three years, except that vocational or technical high schools range from two to four years. Because of a very specialized curriculum, graduates of vocational and technical middle schools are not permitted to enter lycee.

Higher education has the same division between universities and advanced technical and vocational schools. The latter are operated either by the Ministry of Education or other ministries for specialized functions. All universities are public institutions founded individually by special acts of Parliament and administered and controlled by councils elected from the teaching staff.[3] Lycee graduates may enter any university or advanced technical school while graduates of vocational and technical secondary schools may only go to advanced schools of the same type. Higher education ranges from two to six years, depending on the course of study.

In summary, preuniversity education in Turkey lasts eleven years, five at the primary and six at the secondary level. In the academic year 1961/62, 70 percent of the primary-school-age population were enrolled, secondary school enrollment was 16.2 percent of the total number of children of that age, and higher education enrollment was 3.3 percent of the persons of appropriate age.

The Functioning of the Turkish Educational System

While some Middle Eastern nations devote as much as 8 percent of their national income to education and the U.S. allocates some 6.5 percent of its income for this purpose, Turkey spends less than 2.5 percent on education. Expenditures for education, which rose from 1.5 percent of the gross national product in 1948 to 2.2 percent in 1962, have been essentially neutralized by the high relative growth rate of the school-age portion of the population and by inflation of the Turkish lira. The actual expenditures for primary education decreased from 210 TL per capita in 1961 to 198 TL in 1963.

In 1960 more than 60 percent of the population was illiterate, and in some provinces the rate was nearly 90 percent. Table 1-2

TABLE 1–2. PERCENTAGE OF LITERACY IN TURKEY, 1960
(*By Selected Provinces*)

Province	% literate	Province	% literate
Istanbul	73.4	Izmir	56.0
Ankara	55.2	Adana	40.5
Erzurum	28.6	Gumusane	27.5
Mus	17.5	Bitlis	16.1
Hakkari	11.5		

Source: Census of population, 1960.

shows that Turkey's most literate province, Istanbul, had a literacy
rate of 73.4 percent in 1960. Hakkari, in the southeastern part of
Turkey, had a literacy rate of 11.5 percent in 1960, a level comparable to the rate of literacy of all Turkey in 1923. One of the most
discouraging trends in recent years has been that literacy has not
kept pace with population growth. Between 1955 and 1960 the
over-all rate of literacy declined from 40.9 percent to 39.5 percent
(Table 1-3) and the literacy of the rural population dropped from
33.7 percent to 30.3 percent.

TABLE 1–3. CHANGES IN LITERACY RATES BETWEEN 1955 AND 1960 IN TURKEY

		% literacy	
		All of Turkey	Rural population
1955	Male	55.8	49.1
	Female	25.5	18.7
	Total	40.9	33.7
1960	Male	53.6	44.5
	Female	24.8	16.4
	Total	39.5	30.3

Literacy of women is particularly neglected. Enrollment figures
show marked discrepancies between sexes. Of those enrolled in
middle schools and lycees only 25 percent are girls; rural elementary schools have 30 percent girls; and urban elementary schools
have 43 percent girls.

Regional disparities in the quality of education are clearly indicated by comparison of the academic preparation of teachers in
East and West. Less than one-fourth of all middle and lycee
teachers are university graduates and these are concentrated in the
western and northwestern provinces. There are provinces in the
southeast where not a single teacher is a university graduate. This
is obviously related both to the lower socioeconomic level of this
region and the generally lower educational standards.

Table 1-4 shows the relative increase in number of students of
various categories using the year 1927–8 as a base. Lycee enrollment increased dramatically, being forty-one times larger in 1960
than in 1927. During the same period, middle-school enrollment

increased nineteen times and primary-school enrollment increased seven times. Vocational and technical enrollment increased forty-six times, a growth which has taken place mainly in the past fifteen years. University enrollment increased fifteen times.

TABLE 1–4. RELATIVE INCREASE IN NUMBER OF STUDENTS AT VARIOUS EDUCATIONAL LEVELS, 1923–60, USING 1927 POPULATION AS BASE UNIT OF 1 AND SHOWING NUMERICAL FACTORS OF INCREASE ABOVE THAT FIGURE

Year	Primary	Middle	Lycee	Schools for teachers	Vocational and techni-cal schools	University
(No. of students in 1927)	425,997	15,135	1,819	5,022	2,332	4,285
1923–4	0.8	0.4	0.7	0.5	1.7	0.7
1927–8	1.0	1.0	1.0	1.0	1.0	1.0
1935–6	1.6	2.9	6.0	0.6	2.5	1.8
1945–6	3.2	3.9	12.0	3.3	20.9	4.5
1955–6	4.7	8.3	17.1	3.5	38.0	8.7
1960–1	6.7	19.4	41.7	4.0[a]	46.5	15.2

[a] 1958–9

By contrast, the rate of enrollment in teachers' schools has remained dangerously low, having had only a four-fold increase during the period from 1927 to 1959.

Because of limited educational facilities at university level, only a small portion of the lycee graduates can be accepted. Therefore, entrance examinations are required. Repeated efforts have been made to limit the number of students. Lycee graduates who feel they have a right to university training but who fail to pass the entrance exams, still try to use devious methods to gain entrance to the universities and are often successful. It used to be a common spectacle to see them demonstrating in the streets, engaging in sit-down or hunger strikes, and finally being admitted by the hundreds into classes already at least twice the size of even the biggest lecture halls in Ankara and Istanbul. Such selection mechanisms necessarily fostered a high failure rate as faculties tried to reduce enrollment. Another evidence of the drive for higher education is the frequency with which students take multiple entrance examinations for schools as diverse as law, medicine, and engineering, in the hope of passing at least one. An attempt several years ago to force students to choose one field, by scheduling all entrance examinations on the same day, was unsuccessful.

Discipline problems have become progressively more serious as students have learned the power of public demonstrations. In 1960–61 there were student walkouts protesting against politically unpopular teachers. Other protests have been staged against high standards of particular courses and examinations, shortage of books, and poor food in university canteens.

Despite the elevated social status which university professors command, there is a serious and growing problem in recruiting and maintaining a high-quality teaching staff. For example, in one of the faculties in Istanbul University, approximately forty professors and assistant professors are responsible for a student body of about eight thousand. Since enrollment in advanced courses is relatively small, this leaves instructors of beginning classes with as many as two to three thousand students. The problems at examination time are obvious, with a major objective being to screen out the students who should never have been admitted. The academic year lasts nine months, but three of those months are entirely devoted to examinations which are mostly oral, a method wasteful of the time of both students and professors.

Since university pay is low and there is a great demand for educated talent outside the university, many of the best potential teachers leave academic life and those who stay in the universities spend a large part of their time working outside. The vast majority hold two or even three jobs. Even so, promotion to senior positions is limited to those who have worked their way up from the bottom of the academic ladder.

Lectures are often no more than a recital of material in a textbook, which may have been written by the professor himself. Even in small classes there is little use of reports, papers, and student participation. Young Western-trained instructors often find it impossible or impractical to transfer modern teaching methods to their own classes. Students who fail final examinations have been permitted to repeat courses as many times as they like—some as many as eleven times.

In the rural and sparsely settled areas education is progressing particularly slowly. Education levels decline with population density (Table 1-5). Geographic isolation thwarts efforts to change traditional patterns of living. Minimal awareness of the benefits of education is coupled with the strong conservatism of traditional religious beliefs. In the provinces where Turkish is not the mother tongue of the large seminomadic groups, the educational problem is compounded. When children are often hungry, tired, and ill, both parents and children tend to reject schooling. There are some provinces where many of the villages have no schools at all.

TABLE 1–5. PERCENTAGE DISTRIBUTION OF LEVEL OF EDUCATION IN TURKEY ACCORDING TO POPULATION DENSITY (1960)

Places of residence	Total %	No educa-tion	Primary school	Second-ary school	Univer-sity	Un-known
Istanbul	100	22.8	48.7	24.2	3.5	0.8
Cities with population exceeding 100,000	100	30.7	53.7	13.2	2.2	0.2
Cities with population 50,000–100,000	100	36.6	53.8	8.6	0.9	0.1
Cities with population less than 50,000	100	64.3	33.2	2.3	0.1	0.1
Total	100	60.1	35.6	3.7	0.3	0.2

In most of Turkey local governments have minimal or no source of raising funds so that the limited basic social services, such as schools, sanitation, public health and welfare, depend on support from the central government. It is increasingly evident that the low levels of literacy and educational opportunity in eastern and rural areas of Turkey contribute directly to the difficulties the central government is having in redistributing physicians, engineers, and other professional manpower more equitably through the country.

In 1924 Professor John Dewey prepared a report at the invitation of the Ministry of Education, in which he pointed out:

The schools should be, through the cooperation of the teachers and the pupils with public health officials and local physicians, the center of activities to combat the prevalent causes of disease. They should be made responsible for the collecting of statistics and other information needed by the Ministries of Commerce and Agriculture. The object is two-fold: on the one hand, to make sure that there is an organ and center for the collection and dissemination of knowledge which is of national benefit (thereby bringing the schools into connection with the life of the community and nation) and on the other hand, to form in their students, intellectual habits which would be useful to the country and prevent their learning and remaining irrevocably idle and useless.

This high objective still remains to be fulfilled.

REFERENCES

1. Nuri, Eren, *Turkey Today—and Tomorrow* (New York, 1963), p. 132.
2. *Turkish Digest*, No. 4, Vol. 2 (March 15, 1966).
3. Constitutional Law, No. 437, Article 120.

2

HEALTH PROBLEMS AND DISEASE PATTERNS

Precise morbidity and mortality data are almost always a by-product of a highly developed medical system. It follows that health information in a developing country with inadequate health services can be expected to be scanty and approximate.

LIMITATIONS OF TURKISH HEALTH DATA

Although Turkey has modern health services available for some segments of the urban population, the more numerous rural population is largely neglected. Almost 70 percent of the population lives in rural areas where vital statistics data and illnesses are seldom reported. The few available medical personnel have little time to devote to reports because of their other responsibilities and also because communications and transportation are difficult.

Even in urban areas doctors and other health personnel attach little importance to reporting vital and health statistics. Since they are not aware of the potential relevance of such data to health activities, it does not seem to them to be worth the trouble.

Birth certificates are especially unreliable for a number of reasons:

1. Sometimes a deceased baby's birth certificate is used for a newborn baby.
2. Parents may delay reporting a birth until they can be sure that the newborn baby is going to live or in order to produce a delay in subsequent military service for males.
3. Many children born of parents who have had only a religious but not a civil marriage ceremony remain unrecorded.

10

Although by no means complete or accurate, the reporting of deaths is generally more reliable than birth records. A death certificate is necessary for burial in cities and towns, though not in villages. The lack of diagnostic facilities, including laboratories, results in inaccurate cause of death and morbidity data. A local health officer may not report cases of infectious disease because this might reflect on his ability to control disease.

For accurate definition of disease patterns in local communities special surveys will be needed. This would also permit investigation of the relationship of environmental, sociocultural, and other ecologic factors to health patterns. Only a few such studies have been done in Turkey.

DEMOGRAPHIC DATA

The first census in Turkey was in 1927, the second in 1935, and, thereafter, they were repeated at five-year intervals. The total population was 24,064,763 in 1955 and 27,754,820 in 1960. The annual increase was 3.1 percent. At this rate the population would double in twenty-five years. The high dependency ratio is shown in Table 2-1 with 41 percent of the population under fifteen years of age.

Inhabited areas in Turkey are divided, according to administrative criteria rather than population size, into cities, towns, subdistricts, and villages. Cities are mainly the administrative centers of the provinces. Towns usually are the administrative centers of

TABLE 2–1. AGE AND SEX DISTRIBUTION OF THE POPULATION OF TURKEY, 1960

Age Groups	Sex					
	Male	Cumulative %	Female	Cumulative %	Total	Cumulative %
0–4	2,180,155	15.4	2,075,706	15.2	4,255,861	15.3
5–9	2,072,538	30.0	1,924,700	29.3	3,997,238	29.7
10–14	1,687,678	41.9	1,486,229	40.3	3,173,907	41.1
15–44	5,857,906	83.2	5,583,700	81.3	11,441,606	82.3
45–64	1,984,706	97.2	1,908,999	95.3	3,857,705	96.1
65 +	388,087	99.8	590,645	99.7	978,732	99.8
Unknown	28,818	100.0	20,953	100.0	49,771	100.0
Total	14,163,888		13,590,932		27,754,820	

Source: Census of Population 1960, State Institute of Statistics, No. 452.

the districts (*kazas*). *Nahiyes*, or subdistricts, generally have large-sized villages as their centers, and villages include all the smaller communities. All towns and cities are considered urban, though some towns and a few cities are small and have the same environmental conditions as typical villages. The progressive urbanization is shown in Table 2-2 with doubling of the urban population in twenty years. The number of villages increased from 34,787 in 1955 to 35,444 in 1960 and average population per village went up from 493 to 533.

TABLE 2–2. URBAN AND RURAL POPULATION IN TURKEY

Type of area	1940		1950		1960	
	No. of people	%	No. of people	%	No. of people	%
Rural	13,411,242	75.5	15,629,356	74.9	18,895,089	68.1
Urban	4,346,249	24.5	5,244,337	25.1	8,859,731	31.9

Source: Census of Population 1960, State Institute of Statistics, No. 452.

MORTALITY DATA

Deaths are reported more reliably than births, except in villages, where both are grossly under-reported. The crude death rate in ten provinces where data were supposed to be relatively good is shown in Table 2-3. The rapid decline in the crude death rate between 1945 and 1963 must be considered in the light of the rapid population growth of these comparatively urban areas with a probable influx of young adults.

TABLE 2–3. CRUDE DEATH RATE IN TEN PROVINCES[a] BY YEARS

Years	Estimated mid-year population	No. of deaths	Crude death rate per 1,000
1945	1,585,435	27,985	17.7
1949	1,788,731	28,301	15.8
1959	3,698,220	48,021	13.0
1961	4,035,312	48,213	11.9
1963	4,393,692	48,532	11.0

Source: Publications of the State Institute of Statistics, Nos. 345, 407, 427, 476.
[a] These provinces are: Adana, Ankara, Bursa, Cankiri, Denizli, Diyarbakir, Isparta, Istanbul, Izmir, Kutahya.

Causes of Death

Heart and vascular diseases are the major causes of death in cities and towns (Table 2-4). There was a marked increase in this category from 1959 to 1963. Pneumonia ranked second as a cause of death, and these deaths mainly occurred in early childhood. The third cause is infectious and other diseases of newborns and early infancy. Tuberculosis dropped from sixth in 1959 to seventh in 1961. Accidents ranked ninth both in 1959 and 1963.

TABLE 2–4. MAJOR CAUSES OF DEATHS IN TURKISH CITIES AND TOWNS (1959–63)

Causes of deaths	Percent to total deaths		
	1959	1961	1963
Cardio-vascular disease	17.5	19.3	21.6
Pneumonia	16.3	18.1	15.6
Diseases of newborn and early infancy	11.1	11.1	10.9
Gastrointestinal disease	10.8	9.0	8.7
Senility	8.2	8.1	7.2
Tuberculosis	6.0	4.8	4.6
Neoplasm	4.9	5.6	5.9
All the others	25.2	24.0	25.3
Total	100.0	100.0	100.0

Source: Publications of the State Institute of Statistics, Nos. 427 and 476.

Infant Mortality Rate

The infant mortality rate has been considered one of the most sensitive indicators of national levels of health.[1] No country-wide figure is available for the infant mortality rate, but several local studies indicate that it is extremely high.

Students from the Ankara School of Public Health conducted a survey on infant deaths in 1959 which covered 137 villages with 133,000 population. The average infant mortality rate was reported to be 165 with individual villages varying from 125 to 253 per thousand live births.[2]

During a tuberculosis prevalence study conducted by the Ankara School of Public Health and the World Health Organization (WHO) in 1962, a random sample of villagers were questioned about mortality in their families. The average infant mortality rate was 167 per thousand live births in the villages and towns of Yozgat Province.[3]

A large-scale inquiry into fertility and attitudes toward family planning in Turkey was conducted in 1963. Information on infant mortality and crude death and birth rates was collected from a random sample of the nation.[4] The over-all crude death rate was 14.7 per thousand population and the crude birth rate was 41.3 per thousand population. The average infant mortality rate was 247 per thousand live births which varied from 158 in the metropolitan areas to 278 in villages.

In 1965 the Ministry of Health began a continuing demographic survey. The major purpose was to provide current, reliable natality and mortality statistics on an annual and regional basis. According to preliminary findings of this survey,[5] the crude death rate was 18 per thousand population, the crude birth rate was 46 per thousand, and the infant mortality rate was 140 per thousand live births in the part of Central Anatolia surveyed.

According to data collected by the State Institute of Statistics at least 41 percent of deaths in cities and towns in 1962 were children of 0–4 years of age.[6] This figure, of course, would have been higher if information on deaths in villages had been available. Table 2-5 shows a comparison of the percentage of deaths among children under five years of age to the total number of deaths in selected countries.

TABLE 2–5. PERCENTAGE OF DEATHS OF CHILDREN UNDER FIVE YEARS OF AGE
TO THE TOTAL NUMBER OF DEATHS IN SELECTED COUNTRIES

Countries	Percentage of deaths of children under five years to total deaths
Turkey	41.6
United Arab Republic	56.1
Peru	52.4
Romania	12.6
Greece	10.9
France	4.1
U.S.A.	6.9
England and Wales	3.7
Denmark	4.9
Sweden	2.7

Source: *Demographic Yearbook 1963, United Nations*, Statistical Office of the United Nations, Department of Economic and Social Affairs, New York, 1964.

The reporting of morbidity in Turkey is even more incomplete and inaccurate than births and deaths. Morbidity statistics mostly come from hospitals and similar health institutions. Because of the lack of regular registration of diseases and deaths, *ad hoc* surveys are the only sources of relatively reliable data and this information obviously applies mainly to the areas surveyed.

Bacterial Respiratory Infections

Tuberculosis

Tuberculosis is a major disease problem because of the low standards of sanitation, poor nutrition, unsuitable housing, and overcrowding in both urban and rural communities. The disease ranks seventh as a cause of death in cities and towns. It has been estimated that death rates exceed 200 per 100,000 population in most areas.[7] Other estimates are that every year 40,000 persons die from tuberculosis[8] and that there are 900,000 cases of active tuberculosis in the country.[7] According to the State Institute of Statistics, 4.6 percent of the total deaths in cities and towns in 1963 were due to tuberculosis.

Efforts to control tuberculosis have been organized by government and voluntary organizations, with the help of WHO and UNICEF. Between 1953 and 1964, forty-four million people were tuberculin tested or retested and fifteen million were vaccinated or revaccinated with BCG.[9] The number of tuberculosis dispensaries has risen from 41 in 1950 to 115 in 1964 and the bed capacity from 3,548 to 12,674.[10]

In 1960, a well-designed study of tuberculosis morbidity in a small area (Topraklik) of the city of Ankara was conducted by the Ankara School of Public Health. Almost 3 percent showed active or suspected tuberculosis and 0.5 percent of the total 11,329 people examined were positive for tubercle bacilli. Another study by the Ankara School of Public Health in an area of the city near Hacettepe Medical Center in 1961 showed that the prevalence of tuberculosis was 2.5 per hundred.[11]

In 1962, a random-sample survey on the distribution and the prevalence of tuberculosis was conducted in Yozgat Province (where tuberculin sensitivity was particularly high) by the Ankara School of Public Health. The prevalence of pulmonary tuberculosis was 2.5 percent in rural areas and 3 percent in district centers.[12]

The annual fatality rate was 4.7 percent of all tuberculosis cases, 14 percent in cavitary cases, and 9 percent in cases with positive sputa. The attack rate of tuberculosis among BCG-vaccinated persons was reported to be 2.5 times less than in the rest of the population.[8]

With an estimated over-all prevalence rate of 2.6, there are at least 815,000 cases[13] of pulmonary tuberculosis requiring treatment and follow-up. With an estimated annual incidence rate of 0.18 percent 58,000 new pulmonary tuberculosis cases can be expected annually.

Diphtheria

Since diphtheria is reported mainly in the cities and towns, its prevalence in villages is unknown. The State Institute of Statistics reported 410 deaths due to diphtheria in urban areas[14] in 1963. The Ministry of Health's figure was 362 for the whole country which undoubtedly represents extreme under-reporting. Table 2–6 shows the reported cases of diphtheria, deaths, and vaccinations between 1945 and 1964.

TABLE 2–6. OFFICIALLY REPORTED NUMBER OF DIPHTHERIA CASES, DEATHS, AND VACCINATIONS IN TURKEY

Years	Cases reported	Deaths reported	Persons vaccinated
1945	834	69	10,691
1949	953	112	79,369
1955	3,460	405	500,860
1959	3,603	483	858,716
1961	4,573	415	1,020,100
1963	3,575	362	1,247,624
1964	2,921	300	—

Sources: Annual Report on the Communicable Diseases of the Turkish Republic, Ministry of Health, *1925–64* (unpublished), Ankara, Turkey.
Yearbook of Medical Statistics of the Ministry of Health and Social Assistance, 1945–55, Dr. Tunca Yusuf, Publication No. 226, Ankara, 1958.

The initial increase in number of cases is probably due to improved reporting but the decline in recent years is less easily explained. The number of vaccinations against diphtheria increased rapidly among the primary-school children in cities and towns and

provinces had programs of mosquito and larva control and quinine treatment.

In 1942, because of wartime difficulties and military movements, malaria increased and the control program was expanded to include 7,500,000 people. There were 1,323,791 patients receiving treatment in 1949, which was 24.4 percent of the total population in the control area. That year the use of insecticides on a wide scale was started and proper drainage in land development was emphasized. The steady improvement up to 1955 is shown in Table 2–8.

TABLE 2–8. RESULTS OF MALARIA SPLEEN SURVEYS FROM 1925 TO 1955 IN TURKEY

Years	Persons examined	% population with malaria by spleen index
1925	25,718	36.0
1930	1,438,044	16.1
1935	2,036,945	18.0
1940	2,445,222	30.1
1945	5,552,487	41.5
1950	4,545,425	7.1
1953	5,231,162	1.4
1955	1,912,645	0.7

Source: Saglik Calismalarinda Kirk Yil, Publication No. 303, the Ministry of Health, Ankara, Turkey.

By 1956, the malaria control program covered 9,500,000 people. WHO then embarked on a world-wide malaria eradication program. In 1957, UNICEF, WHO, and the Turkish government signed an agreement under which UNICEF contributed supplies, WHO provided technical assistance, and Turkey provided the local budget and personnel. Identification of a case now required detection of parasites in a blood smear. In 1957, 5,536 confirmed cases were detected throughout the country. The next year the number doubled because the local anopheles vector was found to have developed resistance to DDT. Of the 11,213 cases, about 6,000 came from Adana Province. When the insecticide was changed to dieldrin, the number of cases fell to 7,305 in 1959, 3,092 in 1960, 3,498 in 1961, and 3,594[15] in 1962.

Malaria was not thought to occur in the southeast mountainous regions of Turkey until 1961 when some 1,000 cases were discovered. Malariologists had not surveyed this area because it was thought that malaria could not be transmitted at altitudes over 1,500 meters (about 5,000 feet). In 1964, there were still 5,081 cases of malaria in Turkey and about 74 percent (3,760 cases) of them were in southeast Anatolia.[9] The poor living conditions and road communications make it difficult for malaria control teams to reach all homes, and especially nomadic family groups, for spraying and obtaining smears.

Venereal Diseases

Before the establishment of the Turkish republic there were an estimated half a million cases of syphilis. Organized efforts to control venereal diseases were started in 1926. In 1930, 115,367 cases of syphilis were reported. The Ministry of Health now has 11 mobile units or teams, 18 dispensaries (in 1959), and 4 hospitals with 305 beds specifically for venereal disease control. Municipalities and local governments also have some venereal disease control activities as part of their health programs. Table 2–9 shows the progressive reduction in reported number of syphilitic cases under treatment from 1935 to 1960. The apparent reduction in cases is probably artificial since increasing numbers are treated by private physicians who do not report to health authorities and usually do not bother to get serological examinations. Twenty years ago there were many cases of neurosyphilis but today there are few. There were 3,379 new cases of syphilis reported in 1961 and 1,075 cases in 1963.

TABLE 2–9. NUMBER OF OFFICIALLY REPORTED SYPHILITIC CASES UNDER
TREATMENT IN TURKEY

Years	Patients under treatment
1935	161,753
1945	122,631
1950	104,491
1955	61,608
1960	38,966

Source: Publication No. 303, The Ministry of Health.

Legal restrictions in venereal disease control are difficult to enforce even in major cities and towns. They include the requirement that persons wishing to marry must undergo a medical examination with suspected cases being examined serologically. Persons who work in restaurants and public bathing establishments must be medically examined every three months. Licensed prostitutes are to be examined twice weekly by a venereal disease specialist or a government doctor.[30]

As in other countries, there are the problems of increased resistance of the gonococcus to antibiotics and increasing nongonorrheal urethritis, especially in males.

Trachoma

Trachoma continues to be a serious public health problem in Turkey. It is endemic in southeastern and southern Anatolia but many cases are scattered throughout the country. A trachoma control program was started in 1925 when two hospitals were opened, one in Malatya and another in Adiyaman where trachoma infection rates were 90–95 percent with many cases of blindness. Now there are 7 trachoma hospitals with 165 beds and 52 trachoma control dispensaries. Table 2–10 shows the increasing number of cases under treatment between 1935 and 1962 and the reduction in prevalence of trachoma even though more cases have been discovered with increasing diagnostic efforts.

Trachoma is one of the chief causes of blindness in Turkey. There were 101,182 blind people (4.2 per thousand) in Turkey according to 1955 census figures. It was estimated that half of these cases were due to trachoma. The prevalence of blindness in

TABLE 2–10. NUMBER OF TRACHOMA CASES UNDER TREATMENT IN TURKEY

Years	No. of patients	% of cases among people examined
1935	34,782	55
1945	44,603	46
1950	63,122	33
1955	41,982	17
1960	41,762	9
1962	104,073	12

Source: Publication No. 303, the Ministry of Health.

the areas where trachoma is endemic is much higher, ranging around 10 per thousand in Mardin, Gaziantep, Urfa, and Adiyaman.

Leprosy

Leprosy is prevalent throughout much of eastern Anatolia. Today eighteen provinces are classified as endemic regions and eight more range from endemic to sporadic. All provinces have sporadic cases. In 1963, only 3,000 cases of leprosy were recorded. However, it was estimated that there were between 20,000 and 25,000[31] leprosy cases in the whole country. In Elazig Province there is a 265-bed leprosy hospital, and in Istanbul there is a 50-bed ward attached to a mental hospital. In eastern and central Anatolia there are eleven active dispensaries. There is also a leprosy institute, for teaching and research purposes, attached to the Ankara Medical School, to which patients are referred for treatment.

Internationally Quarantinable Diseases

Serious epidemics of cholera have occurred in Turkey within the present century, but no cases have been reported since the end of World War I. Starting in 1912, severe outbreaks occurred and during the war[32] there were at least 30,000 deaths from cholera with more than 10,000 deaths in the Turkish army. The spread of cholera from the Far East to the Middle East in the 1960's has led to intensive diagnostic and immunization programs to prevent introduction from neighboring countries.

In the nineteenth century the territory of the Ottoman Empire was devastated by recurrent plague epidemics. In 1811, the disease spread from Izmir to Istanbul and killed from 500 to 2,000 people daily.[33] After World War I, when the port of Istanbul was occupied by enemy forces, control measures became lax and plague spread through the port area, killing hundreds. Strict control measures have since then limited infection to only occasional cases[34] and since 1947 no cases have been reported.

Smallpox vaccination has been compulsory in Turkey since 1915.[35] However, because of inadequate organization and personnel, localized outbreaks of smallpox have continued to occur, particularly in the eastern and southern provinces. In 1924 a severe form of the disease was introduced from Iraq and attained a maximum of 1,746 cases[36] in 1929. In 1942 smallpox recurred in the border provinces of Mardin and Urfa and spread through Anatolia to European Turkey with recorded cases increasing from 1,871 in 1942 to 12,395 in 1943. Widespread vaccination resulted in reduction of reported cases from 6,093 in 1944 to 309 in 1945[21] and only 10 cases in 1946. No cases have been reported since 1958 but there is always the danger of the disease being imported.

Severe typhus epidemics attacked both the military and civilian population of Turkey between 1913 and 1922. Although there were localized outbreaks after that, no major epidemics occurred until 1943 when 4,142 cases were recorded. Vigorous control measures included mass immunization and DDT spraying of affected groups. Incidence then showed a continuous decline from 394 cases in 1948 to 225 cases in 1950, 24 cases in 1957, and 7 cases in 1958.[37] There were 5 cases in 1961, 10 cases in 1962, and 1 case each in 1963 and 1964.[36]

Only a few cases of relapsing fever have been reported, with three cases in 1950 and one in 1952.

GENERAL STATE OF ENVIRONMENTAL SANITATION IN TURKEY

Turkey does not have a strong environmental sanitation control organization. The Ministry of Health includes within its General Directorate of Health a Division of Environmental Sanitation which is supposed to be concerned with food, milk, municipal water supply, excreta disposal, nuisances, hotels, bathing places, and zoning for factories. This division has little direct responsibility or authority and the personnel do scarcely more than handle correspondence with other agencies and keep records.

The actual enforcement of regulations relating to sanitation is the responsibility of municipal health departments in bigger cities and medical officers of health in towns and rural areas. *Saglik memurus* are expected to do most of the actual control work under the supervision of municipality doctors and medical officers of health. Each of these individuals, however, has many other responsibilities in public medical care services, legal medicine, and collecting statistical data. Many of them devote their major attention to their own private practice after working hours. Not only are they unable to give enough time to public health duties but, even more important, they have had little training in environmental health.

Many of the major health problems in Turkey are related to sanitation. Rates of tuberculosis are affected by housing; malaria, by water drainage; typhoid fever, dysentery, parasitism, and ancylostomiasis, by excreta disposal; and brucellosis, by milk sanitation. Human comfort, personal cleanliness, and community pride are important ingredients of individual and group efforts to improve sanitation.

Only 510 of the 1,053 municipalities in Turkey have piped water supply. Of the 63,805* village communities, 25,775 have no piped water supply, 16,700 have pipelines providing insufficient water which is likely to be contaminated, and only 21,330 have piped water supply sufficient for present needs. Of 12,543 drinking water samples examined bacteriologically in the Central Laboratory during 1963 and 1964, 5,568 were contaminated.

There is not a city, town, or village in Turkey which has a properly designed sewage disposal system. Pollution of water sources and gross soil contamination are the result. In rural areas, the surface method of excreta disposal promotes fly breeding. Urban refuse collection and disposal is similarly primitive. Gypsies pick over open refuse bins in domestic areas and their salvage finds its way back into the market in much the same form as it was retrieved from the bin.

On the outskirts of large cities a fringe development of *gecekondu* (overnight houses) is taking place. Shacks are put up overnight on appropriated land by the large number of people crowding into cities. Such encroachment results in unsanitary pit privies, contaminated shallow wells, and poorly-cared-for animals. Additional heavy government expenditure will be required to provide any type of sanitation service under these conditions.

Contamination of vegetables by human excreta which is used as fertilizer is particularly dangerous because much of the produce is eaten raw. Restaurants and hotels are regularly inspected by health officials but inspections tend to become casual visits and only grossly unhygienic conditions are reported. The slaughterhouses in municipalities vary from modern and well-equipped abattoirs to small timber sheds with concrete floors. They are supposed to be controlled by veterinarians.

---

*These village communities are administered by 35,444 *muhtars*. Therefore, the total number of villages is much larger than the number quoted in the section on midwives in Chapter 5.

General nutritional status is influenced by a wide range of economic, medical, agricultural, political, hygienic, religious, and social factors. Local food consumption is determined by family feeding habits and climatic and agricultural conditions. Variations are marked in the different parts of Turkey, between towns and villages and from season to season.[38]

The Turkish Diet

The main food is *bread*. Generally made from whole wheat or rye, it is the basic staple for the entire country providing 50 to 60 percent of total calories. Another wheat product, *bulgur*, is used extensively in villages. It is made by boiling wheat in water for sixty to ninety minutes and then drying it in the sun before it is hulled and cracked. Meat is not generally available. In some coastal regions fresh and dried fish are a cheap and plentiful source of protein for both rich and poor. Eggs are eaten only during seasons when they are cheap. In summary, most of the nourishment in the Turkish diet is provided by carbohydrates.

A few studies have been done on the quality and quantity of diets during various seasons. These studies[38] showed that "peasant's winter meals" provide about 70 percent of "safe practical allowances" of caloric value of protein food as measured in NDpCals percent (Net Dietary–protein calories percent) for toddlers and adolescents, but do not meet the "minimum" protein requirement for lactating mothers. "Peasant's summer meals" and "middle-class winter meals" are somewhat better but still not up to the level of "safe practical allowances" for toddlers, adolescents, and lactating mothers. The "middle-class summer meals" do meet "safe practical allowances" of NDpCals percent for toddlers and adolescents but not for lactating mothers. Each of these diets provided an appropriate protein balance for adults and children but the quantity of food was not sufficient to meet the basic standards used in the study.

Infant diets are even more grossly deficient. They are far below even the minimum requirements of NDpCals percent, providing only 4 percent of NDpCals. Prepared baby foods available in Turkey are made mainly from starch. Even after 15 percent whole milk powder was added, they did not contain enough protein. As recommended by a FAO committee,[39] both the quality and quantity of protein supplements must be improved.

These comparisons indicate that the Turkish diet must be supplemented with protein-rich foods to meet standard nutritional levels. The lack is particularly great among the poor and the very young.

ICNND Survey of Armed Forces

A nutritional survey of the Turkish armed forces was conducted under the auspices of the Interdepartmental Committee on Nutrition for National Defense (ICNND),[40] during the spring of 1957. Clinical examinations were conducted on a total of 8,519 Turkish soldiers, sailors, and airmen (1,707 detailed examinations and 6,812 screening tests) with biochemical analysis of urine and blood. Dietary intake studies were done in kitchens feeding approximately 8,000 men per day. The findings of the survey indicated that in general the nutritional status of the Turkish armed forces was good, with adequate calories, protein, iron, calcium, thiamin, and niacin. But the margin of safety in other nutrients narrowed, with a borderline supply of vitamin C, vitamin A, and riboflavin.

Malnutrition in the General Population

Malnutrition is a significant health problem in Turkey. Nutritional deficiencies are responsible for many of the deaths recorded as gastrointestinal or lower respiratory infections or childhood exanthemata. This synergism has been extensively studied in recent years in Guatemala, India, and elsewhere.[41]

Turkey fits the general pattern of developing countries where "the weaning syndrome" is the first cause of death. About half of all deaths occur in children below five. In the past these fatalities have been ascribed to the infection which served as the obvious final cause of death: the common diarrheas, respiratory infections, and childhood exanthemata such as measles. These infections are not ordinarily fatal in well-nourished individuals. The cycle of deterioration of health leading to death follows a clear sequence: the child is in a borderline nutritional state as a result of the rapid shift from breast feeding to adult diet at weaning; acute infections are picked up as a normal part of the early explorations of the toddler; the infection directly causes deterioration of the nutritional status with marked loss of protein; nutritional deficiencies are known to cause sharp reduction in the body's defenses against infection so that more severe infections supervene; progressive malnutrition with incipient or actual *kwashiorkor* or marasmus leads to an eventually fatal infection.

According to observations at Hacettepe Medical Center,[42] the majority of children are within the normal weight range during the early months of life when they are breast fed. Then large numbers develop signs of malnutrition as they are weaned with no additional milk or food supplement other than cereal gruels and starch water. According to research done in Izmir,[43] 37.6 percent of babies are breast fed beyond the first three months, 21 percent beyond one year, and 13 percent beyond fifteen months. In rural Turkey breast feeding is continued as long as possible and the shift to cereal gruels and starch water occurs only as breast milk becomes insufficient. Turkish villagers drink very little cow's milk. Since much of the milk is contaminated, it is easy to see why. Frequently, infants brought to Hacettepe hospital have been living on starch water for as long as six months.

Turkish parents rarely bring their children to physicians because of malnutrition. Malnutrition develops slowly and insidiously and parents are often not aware that a problem exists, especially since babies are swaddled and a quiet child is considered a good child. The parents wait until secondary infection produces symptoms which they recognize as illness. Then they bring the child to the doctor with major complications such as dysentery, dehydration, acidosis, and pneumonia.

In health statistics, also, estimates of morbidity and mortality from malnutrition are not available because the cause of the disease is usually attributed to an associated infection. One report estimates that malnutrition is responsible for 35 to 40 percent of all deaths.[43] The high fatality rate from measles, bronchopneumonia, and infant diarrhea is certainly related to malnutrition. The high rate of pulmonary tuberculosis among adolescents is also partly due to malnutrition.

Once malnutrition has developed, treatment is expensive and time-consuming. The solution to the problem is prevention and this requires health education and an expanded maternal and child health program.

THE RATE OF POPULATION GROWTH

The greatest public health problem of Turkey today is its high rate of population growth. The lag between the fall in death rate and the birth rate, which is typical of a rapidly developing country, leads directly to the present transitional situation with the population increasing by about 3 percent per year, or doubling in approximately one generation. The critical necessity is to shorten the period of demographic transition as much as possible by the many measures needed to create the preconditions for a prompt reduction in the birth rate. Family planning must be made an important part of the general health program.

The most obvious health implication of the rapid rate of population increase is the difficulty of maintaining expansion of health services along with education and all the other benefits of civilized society to match the increasing numbers. This is clearly brought out in the chapter "Projection of Demand," where minimum calculations consistently show the need for rapidly expanding manpower just to maintain status quo ratios. Even more specific health complications of excess fertility are being increasingly defined. It is now known from studies in other developing countries that high parity and short interpregnancy intervals cause increased maternal mortality, neonatal mortality, infant mortality, and childhood mortality under two years of age.[43] Even more pervasive is the general finding that in a large family, sibling competition for food and the mother's care has a generally negative effect on the health of children and on their future development.

With the recent recognition of the primary importance of population growth[5] in Turkey, a national population program has been started. The Ministry of Health has been made responsible and pilot projects and studies have been started. A major investment of health manpower will be needed in this new and important activity.

SUMMARY

Turkey has a population of 27,754,820 according to the 1960 census, with a rate of population growth of 3 percent per year. The birth rate is 47.7 per 1,000 population, whereas the death rate has dropped to 10.9 per 1,000.

Turkey's population still suffers, however, from a wide variety of infectious diseases. These can be reduced if improved nutrition, housing, environmental sanitation, and preventive and public health services are more widely available. Much progress in the health field has resulted from control of major epidemic diseases such as smallpox, cholera, plague, typhus fever, and malaria. However, much more intensive work must be done before tuberculosis, leprosy, trachoma, diarrheal and dysentery diseases, and the many common childhood diseases are under adequate control.

The health status of Turkey resembles that of the United States sixty years ago. With the ambitious public health, preventive medicine, and community development programs underway in Turkey, one can optimistically look forward to an enormous reduction of "preventable disease" in this decade. The Turkish government has made major commitments to this end through the Nationalized Health Service which was started in 1963.

References

1. *Measurement of Levels of Health*, WHO Technical Report Series No. 137, WHO—Geneva, 1957.
2. "Orta ve Bati Anadoluda 137 Koyde Ana ve Cocuk Dogum ve Olumleri Uzerinde Yapilan Etud Sonuclari," Ankara Hifzissihha Okulu (Ankara School of Public Health) August, 1959. (Unpublished.)
3. "Yozgat Tuberkuloz Prevalans Calismasinda Ornekleme ile Secilen Hanelerde Bir Yillik Ara ile Yapilan Ev Halki Tespit ve Kontrollari Sonucu," Ankara Hifzissihha Okulu, 1962. (Unpublished.)
4. K. E. Gales, "The Report of an Inquiry into Birth and Death Rates in Turkey," Ankara, 1963. (Unpublished.)
5. N. Fisek, Y. Heperkan, and J. Rumford, "The Evolution of the Turkish Demographic Survey," (Ministry of Health and Social Assistance, Ankara, January, 1966). (Unpublished.)
6. N. Fisek, Y. Heperkan, and J. Rumford, "The Role of the Turkish Demographic Survey in the Family Planning and Rural Health Programs," Ankara, 1963. (Unpublished.)
7. *Medico-Sosyal Saglik Dergisi*, Vol. 31 (July, 1965), p. 46.
8. "Report on the Activities of Tuberculosis Training and Research Department of the Ankara School of Public Health, 1959–64." (Unpublished, Ankara.)
9. *T. C. Saglik ve Sosyal Yardim Bakanligi 1965 Calismalari* (Ankara, 1965), p. 5.
10. "Number of Health Institutions and Their Bed Capacity in Turkey" (JHU Health Manpower Project in Turkey—Draft, 1965). (Unpublished.)
11. *Studies on Hacettepe and Topraklik Prevalence Surveys* (Ankara School of Public Health, 1961).
12. *A Tuberculosis Prevalence Survey in Turkey* (Ankara School of Public Health, 1964), p. 13.
13. *Preliminary Results of 1965 Population Census*, Publ. No. 484, State Institute of Statistics, Ankara, 1966.
14. *Il ve ilce Merkezlerinde Olumler 1963*, T. C. Basbakanlik Devlet Istatistik Enstitusu Baskanligi Yayin No. 476.
15. *Saglik Calismalarinda Kirk Yil*, Ministry of Health Publication No. 303, Ankara.
16. Ceyhun A. Kansu, "Infant Mortality in Turkish Villages," *The Turkish Journal of Pediatrics*, Vol. 3 (1961).
17. Simmons, Whayne, Anderson, and Horack, *Global Epidemiology*, Vol. 3 (1951), pp. 205–32.

18. "Shigellosis—A Preventive Medicine Problem in Turkey," Tuslog Det. 36 APO (1963), pp. 63–67.
19. N. Fisek and N. Akyay, "The Control of Typhoid and Paratyphoid Fevers in Turkey," *Turkish Bulletin of Hygiene and Experimental Biology*, Vol. 14, No. 3 (1956).
20. Personal interview with Dr. Erel, D. and Dr. Sellioglu, B.
21. Personal interview with Dr. Akyol Muzaffer.
22. "Report on Intestinal Parasites among Primary School Children" (The Ankara School of Public Health). (Unpublished.)
23. Personal interview with Dr. Akalin, B.
24. "Intestinal Ova and Parasite Survey of Indigenous Food Handlers—Turkey," Tuslog Det. 36 APO (1963), pp. 63–65.
25. Dr. Ari, A. "Polio Vaccination Campaign in Turkey," *Saglik Dergisi*, Vol. 37 (1964), pp. 3–4.
26. Dr. Ari, A. article in *Turkish Bulletin of Hygiene and Experimental Biology*, Vol. 24, No. 2 (1964).
27. Dr. Akyol, M. "The Actual Situation of Infectious Diseases in Turkey" (1965). (Unpublished), Ankara.
28. Dr. Erginoz, H."Evaluation of the Activities on Measles in Ankara Province," Unpublished. Diploma of Public Health Dissertation, 1965.
29. *Mediko-sosyal Saglik Dergisi* (Jan. 1965), p. 42.
30. Sven Christiansen, "Report of Syphilis Control in Turkey," *WHO Bulletin* Vol. 10 (1954), pp. 627–90.
31. Dr. B. Cvjetanovic, "Report on a Visit to Turkey," WHO Report, 1956. (Unpublished.)
32. Abdulkadir Noyan, *Son Harplerde Salgin Hastalkiklarla Savaslarim*, Tip Fakultesi Yayinlari, Vol. 54 (1956), p. 9.
33. Osman Sevki, *Vebanin Memleketimizde Tarihi* (Askeri Tip Mecmuasi, 1919), pp. 28–30.
34. Zuhtu Berke, *Turkish Bulletin of Hygiene and Experimental Biology, Vol. 14* (1954), p. 3.
35. *Telkihi Cudre Nizamnamesi Madde*, No. 19 (Sept. 30, 1915).
36. "Annual Report on the Communicable Diseases of the Turkish Republic" (Ministry of Health, 1925–64). (Unpublished.)
37. United Nations, *Demographic Yearbook 1963* (New York, 1964).
38. Dr. Orhan Koksal, Abstract of thesis submitted for degree of Master of Science in Nutrition, University of London.
39. F.A.O. Nutritional Studies No. 16 (1957).
40. Z. I. Kertesz, *Food Technology Survey in Turkey: Nutrition Survey of the Armed Forces*, "Part IV, Interdepartmental Committee on Nutrition for National Defense, U.S.A." (1957).
41. Anne Burgess and R. F. A. Dean (eds.), *Malnutrition and Food Habits* (Tavistock Publications, London, 1962), pp. 29–37.
42. I. Dogramaci and T. D. Wray, "Severe Infantile Malnutrition and Its Management," *The Turkish Journal of Pediatrics*, Vol. 1 (1965).
43. S. Cura, "The Social Aspects of Child Nutrition in Turkey," *The Turkish Journal of Pediatrics* (1961), p. 3.

3

THE DOCTOR IN TURKEY—SUPPLY AND DYNAMICS OF PROFESSIONAL RELATIONSHIPS

Like many other nations, Turkey had no accurate information on the number of doctors in the country or their distribution. Although many doctors were known to have left Turkey, no one knew how many. The registration lists of the Ministry of Health were not up-to-date. Most doctors were registered at the time of graduation but many on the list were deceased. Also, some doctors who were actively practicing in Turkey were not registered. A basic census was necessary before any other studies of doctors could be undertaken.

This section includes four studies in addition to the "Census of Doctors." A 10 percent sample of all doctors was studied in detail to define the "Professional Problems of Doctors." "The Doctor's Role in the Private Sector" required a separate study. "Attitudes Toward Rural Service" were studied in four sample groups using a specially adapted battery of tests. "A Crisis in Medical Education" is a report of direct observation of present teaching techniques, curriculum, cost of education, and educational trends.

CENSUS OF DOCTORS

A verified count of doctors provides the foundation on which a health manpower study can be built. Planning of both medical care and public health services requires as a first step knowledge of the available supply of physicians, their ages, present activity status, type of work, and geographical distribution.

This census was limited to doctors who graduated between 1923 and 1963. It is difficult and unnecessary to trace doctors who have already retired. In Turkish government service retirement age is sixty-five and doctors who graduated in 1923 would have reached this age by 1963. Reasonable extrapolations could be made on doctors in private practice.

Materials and Methods

The sources of information and procedure for data collection included:

1. Combined lists of all the graduates of the three Turkish medical schools up to 1963. A second basic list was obtained from the registration books of the Ministry of Health where all graduates, including those who had studied abroad, were supposed to be registered. Cross-checking showed that 3 percent of doctors practicing in Turkey were not registered with the Ministry of Health, as required by law. Conversely, the medical school lists failed to include the names of some graduates, mainly army doctors, who had not paid diploma fees.

2. Address lists of three pharmaceutical companies—the Eczacibasi, Bayer, and Ibrahim Ethem laboratories. Their co-operation was obtained by promising them the final corrected lists of doctors for their own use. When these corrected lists were sent, the firms were asked to report new addresses to the registry in the future.

3. Address lists of all doctors who were working in the Ministry of Health. These were obtained to get current information on their location.

4. An inventory questionnaire sent to all public and private institutions. This was utilized to get information on doctors as well as other health personnel. Answers included the names and addresses of doctors, schools and dates of graduation, and present activities. These were checked against information from other sources.

5. A monthly medical bulletin called *Dirim*, published by Dr. Feridun Frik. This bulletin listed most of the deaths of doctors. All officially notified deaths are recorded in a special Ministry of Health registration book. When these two sources were cross-checked, it was found that the Ministry's records on deaths were very poor. Until a new approach is used, the Ministry's death registration book will serve little purpose.

6. Interviews with groups of doctors from each graduation year of all medical schools. These were necessary to check surnames and present addresses of former classmates. The surname was legally required for the first time in Turkey in 1934. Prior to that, first names were listed without surnames and this change created serious difficulties. The graduates of each class were asked to match the graduation names of their friends with present names and to provide current information. A similar procedure was used to obtain names and addresses of female physicians whose surnames were changed by marriage.

7. Inquiries to the German Embassy and the German Medical Chamber. Information about Turkish doctors in Germany was requested, but no answers were received.

8. The "Thank You Notes for Doctors" which are traditionally printed in newspapers by grateful patients. These yielded names and addresses of doctors.

From the above sources, a composite list was prepared of Turkish doctors according to year of graduation (Table 3–1). A second list recorded them alphabetically by surname. This listing was the first of its kind in Turkey and serves as the basis for a revised registration system with a complete card file on all doctors.

A simple one-page questionnaire was prepared and sent to all physicians working in Turkey whose addresses were available. The questions covered professional status, present employment (including multiple employment), income, experience, and past

TABLE 3–1. NUMBER OF TURKISH[a] GRADUATES FROM TURKISH MEDICAL SCHOOLS
BY YEAR OF GRADUATION

Year of graduation	Name of medical school			
	Istanbul	Ankara	Izmir	Total
1923–9	549	—	—	549
1930–9	1,409	—	—	1,409
1940–9	3,535	462	—	3,997
1950–9	3,332	1,580	—	4,912
1960–3	1,087	536	197	1,820
Total	9,912	2,578	197	12,687
Percent	78.1	20.3	1.6	100.0

[a] 578 foreign graduates are not included.

and proposed trips to other countries. The questionnaire was short, easy to fill out, and had a stamped, self-addressed envelope. Questionnaires were not sent to doctors known to be abroad since this census was only for doctors living in Turkey.

The first mailing was of 10,150 questionnaires between March 16 and May 4, 1964. Later 912 more addresses were found and the number of questionnaires mailed increased to 11,062. Respondents to the first mailing totaled 4,701. To those who did not respond six different reminders were sent up to October, 1964. The number of doctors who finally responded was 7,418.

Findings

Total Number of Doctors

From the medical school records it was estimated that 12,875 Turkish doctors had graduated from Turkish and foreign medical schools between 1923 and 1963, of whom 10,027 were estimated to be available in Turkey in 1964 as a manpower pool (Table 3–2). In the census returns, 403 deaths were definitely reported. Extrapolation of the findings of the subsequent 10 percent sample study suggested that a further 200 deaths were probable, so that estimated total deaths were 600. Extrapolation from the detailed sample study findings also provided an estimate of 2,248 Turkish doctors who were abroad.

TABLE 3–2. NUMBER OF TURKISH DOCTORS GRADUATED (1923–63)

Number of graduates from Turkish medical schools	12,687
Number of graduates from foreign medical schools	188
Total	12,875
Estimated number of deaths	600
Estimated to be abroad	2,248
Available supply of doctors	10,027

It was estimated that not more than 200 doctors who graduated prior to 1923 may still have been alive in 1963. They were probably not very active, even in private practice. The figure of 200 was calculated by applying the death rate average of 1923–5 graduates to the number of graduates with an upward adjustment to take into consideration the higher death rate of 1913–23 graduates and also the typhus epidemic during World War I which had a high fatality rate among doctors.

A recent book[1] by Dr. Feridun Frik presents the independent estimate of 10,948 as being the number of doctors practicing in Turkey in 1963. Dr. Frik's estimate was based on data gathered mostly by the sales representatives of a German drug firm who were developing a complete list of potential clientele. The addresses of these doctors were supplied by Dr. Frik, but the postal service returned 614 questionnaires with notes indicating that they were either abroad or deceased. By subtracting this number and also the estimated 200 who may have graduated prior to 1923, the number is reduced to 10,134. The difference between Dr. Frik's figure and ours then is only 107. This small difference might be due to changes which occurred during the interval between the studies or because of minor inaccuracies in estimates.

Of the 10,027 Turkish doctors, 7,418 or 74 percent responded to the mailed questionnaire for the doctor's census. This is considered a favorable response rate for a mailed questionnaire, especially in view of the question dealing with income which will be discussed later.

Distribution of Doctors

The distribution of doctors is important because of known geographical inequalities in health services. The number of doctors in each province was extrapolated from the 7,418 respondents to the 10,027 total estimate. These figures were checked against Dr. Frik's lists for each province and found to be close.

The simplest analysis of the distribution of doctors in Turkey is to calculate the doctor/population ratios in each of the eight regions (Table 3-3). The Black Sea coast and southeastern and eastern Anatolia have the fewest doctors and the European and Central Anatolian regions have the most. Regional grouping disguises further maldistributions. Whereas, 6,450 doctors (64.5 percent) were working in three provinces (namely, Ankara, Istanbul, and Izmir) which represent only 15.8 percent of the total population, 2,947 doctors (29.5 percent) were serving the 56.2 percent of the total population in thirty-nine provinces and 603 doctors (6 percent) were practicing in twenty-five provinces which had 28 percent of the total population.

Some Professional Characteristics

Of the 7,418 respondents, 1,944 (26.2 percent) were general practitioners, 4,542 (61.2 percent) were specialists, and 910 (12.3

TABLE 3–3. DISTRIBUTION OF TURKISH DOCTORS AND POPULATION BY REGION (1964)

Region	Estimated 1964 population	Number of doctors	Number of persons per doctor
Turkey in Europe	3,006,000	3,948	761
Black Sea coast	4,907,000	555	8,841
Marmara and Aegean Sea coasts	4,933,000	1,462	3,373
Mediterranean Sea coast	2,336,000	473	4,938
West Anatolia	2,590,000	391	6,623
Central Anatolia	7,594,000	2,561	2,965
Southeast Anatolia	1,317,000	159	8,284
East Anatolia	3,946,000	451	8,749
Total	30,629,000	10,000	3,063

percent) were in specialty training. Only 22 (0.3 percent) of the doctors did not give information about specialization.

Because of the known importance of emigration, doctors were asked if they had been or planned to go abroad. Four percent of general practitioners and 25 percent of specialists or residents had already been abroad. Twenty percent of general practitioners and 22 percent of specialists or residents planned to go abroad in 1964.

It was expected that doctors going abroad would be mainly recent graduates, but this did not prove to be true (Table 3–4). A fairly

TABLE 3–4. DISTRIBUTION OF TURKISH DOCTORS WHO HAVE OR HAVE NOT PLANNED TO GO ABROAD TO WORK, BY YEAR OF GRADUATION

Year of graduation	Total no. of respondents	Have no plans		Have plans	
		No.	%	No.	%
1923–45	2,476	2,109	85.2	367	14.8
1946–50	1,471	1,145	77.9	326	22.1
1951–4	1,211	878	72.5	333	27.5
1955–9	1,189	863	72.6	326	27.4
1960–3	1,049	805	76.8	244	23.2
Total[a]	7,396	5,800	78.4	1,596	21.6

[a] Twenty-two doctors did not give information on their plans.

uniform percentage of graduates leaving school since World War
II are making plans to go abroad. This must mean that travel overseas is not necessarily for specialist training and that dissatisfaction
with practice in Turkey is not limited to young doctors. The 1960–
3 group of graduates shows a slightly lower percentage than
previous years, probably because many graduates have to complete
their compulsory military service before going ahead with other
plans.

That doctors were planning to go abroad to work rather than to
receive advanced training was further confirmed by their choice of
foreign countries (Table 3–5). Many of them were going to West
Germany where the employment opportunities were particularly
good for general practitioners.

TABLE 3–5. FOREIGN COUNTRIES TO WHICH TURKISH DOCTORS PLANNED TO GO IN 1964

| Specialty | Total respon- dents | Doctors having plans | % of total | Foreign Countries | | |
				U.S.	West Germany	Others
General practitioners	1,944	389	20.0	61	215	113
Specialists or residents	5,452	1,207	22.1	261	530	416
Total	7,396	1,596	21.6	322	745	529

Although doctors' income is discussed in detail in the next section, special consideration of the income of doctors planning to go
abroad is relevant here. It is probable that better financial remuneration is one consideration since doctors with lower incomes
showed a somewhat greater inclination to leave Turkey (Table 3–6).

Conducting a census proved time-consuming and expensive, but
it was a necessary and productive part of this health manpower
study. Subsequent detailed sample studies required an accurate
list of all the doctors in Turkey. Deficiencies were identified in the
recording systems of both the Ministry of Health and the medical
schools and a new registry based on a complete card file was started.
The census also provided indications of areas needing further study
and of doctors' attitudes toward certain types of questions. For instance, it became clear that the response rate would have been
higher if we had not asked a direct question about doctor's income.

TABLE 3–6. TOTAL MONTHLY INCOME OF DOCTORS WHO PLANNED TO GO
ABROAD, IN 1964

Total monthly income (T.L.)	No. of doctors who responded	Have plans to go abroad	
		No.	%
999 or less	1,205	298	24.7
1000–1999	2,096	527	25.1
2000–2999	1,896	400	21.1
3000 or more	2,004	336	16.7
No answer or unknown	195	35	18.6
Total	7,396	1,596	21.6

PROFESSIONAL PROBLEMS OF DOCTORS

Most Turkish doctors are unhappy. They say that their professional frustrations are numerous and cumulative. The current situation is in marked contrast to the long history of high social prestige and official status accorded to doctors in Turkey. For manpower planning, it is essential to find out if the present problems and future prospects are as claimed.

Behind most of the professional problems lies a fundamental social tension. Traditional goals and personal desires of the medical profession have created a strong trend toward hospital-oriented specialization and urban concentration while the growing pressures of national needs require the development of comprehensive health services for rural areas. Such apparent incompatibilities between professional goals and social objectives make doctors feel that medical practice is being forced into patterns which are contrary to their understanding of the role of physicians. Doctors are, therefore, resorting to a variety of escape devices to avoid politically imposed requirements and restrictions.

Simply stated, most of the immediate problems result from the inability of present manpower resources to meet a suddenly expanding demand. In the past, scientific medical care was available only for the upper classes who were sufficiently affluent to make medical practice lucrative. As a result of the social revolution of the past generation the common people are beginning to view health benefits as a fundamental right. The demand is further augmented by accelerating population growth. Political promises of improved health services for everyone have been generally publicized. The economic justification that healthy citizens will be more productive citizens supports the well-recognized vote-getting potential of promised health services.

It is time for the medical profession to take the leadership in finding equitable and reasonable solutions for the increasingly evident deficiencies. Medical leaders are, in fact, becoming more and more concerned about ethical implications of the unmet health needs and are eager to apply scientific principles to the search for better ways of improving health services.

Two major limitations are apparent; the first is financial and the second administrative. The money available for health services, both from private and public sources, is so little that many doctors have great difficulty in earning a reasonable living wage, so merely planning for more doctors is not the answer. The only possibility of meeting the rising popular demand is to think innovatively about major administrative reorganization and to develop new ways of making more efficient use of the limited numbers of professionals.

The observation that young medical graduates are pessimistic about their professional future recurs at many points throughout this analysis. It underlies the efforts of doctors to escape the service requirements imposed on them by society. They have doubts about their ability to undertake independent responsibility under the difficult and pioneering conditions of the rural health services where they are most obviously needed. This insecurity partially explains the trend toward specialization, urban concentration, and emigration to more developed countries. Among the practical generalizations to be derived from such findings are the clear requirements for the new nationalization program to provide the right kind of professional support for young doctors in peripheral units and for a new pattern of medical education to prepare doctors for their new responsibilities.

An intensive study was done to explore in depth the following specific issues: the number of doctors holding more than one job; the income levels of doctors; their attitudes toward private practice; doctor's attitudes about the plan for nationalization of health services; the problems of the public health officer; urban concentration; the degree to which medical education is subsidized by government scholarships; distribution of general practitioners and specialists; the high rate of specialization; the escape of doctors from Turkey to foreign countries; doctors not now in practice; and their advice to their own children about health careers.

Materials and Methods

A random sample of approximately 10 percent of all living Turkish doctors who graduated between 1923–63 was drawn. Because of the importance of the fundamental issues being investigated, a concentrated effort was made to get a complete response from all the doctors in the sample. This was especially difficult because the complexity of the forms required a high level of co-operation. With a great investment of time and money, the unusually high response rate of 97.2 percent of the sample was achieved. (This was in contrast to a response rate of 74 percent from the general census of doctors.)

Sampling Design

The sampling universe for this investigation included all Turkish graduates from 1923–63 excluding those known to be dead. The names were listed alphabetically by surnames. If a doctor did not have a surname,* his given name was listed. Information on address, date of birth, date of graduation, and related data was recorded on a separate card for each doctor. Using a table of random numbers, 1,257 doctors were selected from the list of 1923–63 graduates of Turkish and foreign medical schools. A reserve sample of fifty was also selected at the same time in order to have replacements for doctors in the sample who might be deceased. Later it was determined that eighteen of the doctors in our sample were dead, and names from the reserve sample were substituted.

Questionnaire Construction, Pre-Testing, and Tracking of Unknown Addresses

The questionnaire was normally administered as a personal interview, but in a small number of cases it was mailed to remote and isolated areas.

A preliminary questionnaire was developed and pretested on 200 doctors not in our sample during the training period of the interviewers. Two questions were eliminated and four others were markedly simplified. Despite this pretesting, an additional question about those daily activities which the doctor considered unrelated

* There were 186 doctors in the sampling universe whose surnames could not be found; all of them were graduates of Istanbul Medical School prior to 1934. In June, 1934, a law was passed which made it obligatory for every person to adopt a distinct surname.

to his professional capacities should have been omitted because the answers proved of no value.

The last question was a request for information from classmates of the doctors who had not yet been located. This proved to be a highly successful tracking method leading to many previously unknown addresses. Another means of obtaining unknown addresses was to send lists of classmates to doctors who had already been located through the census study. In order to gain maximum cooperation an extra list of all known addresses of each doctor's classmates was included for the respondent's personal interest. They were asked to return one copy of this list with the addition of any addresses known to them. This method was most successful in tracing doctors who had emigrated or died.

A simple but important method for tracing doctors in the sample was a special search of the records of the Ministry of Health. When employed by the Ministry, a doctor names a beneficiary in case of sudden or unexpected death. Physicians whose addresses were unknown were located by writing to the relatives or friends indicated in these records. This method was most useful in finding doctors who were abroad or who had returned to Turkey after having been abroad for many years.

The effectiveness of these methods is indicated by the fact that 240 doctors, for whom we had no clues about location, were traced to their residence if living or to definite information that they were dead. This left only 14 doctors from the original sample about whom no information could be obtained.

Data Collection

Each doctor's address was identified on a map of Turkey. The distribution in the sample was essentially the same as the general distribution of doctors in Turkey.

For the direct interviews, Turkey was divided into seven regions on the basis of accessibility to transportation facilities and cost of travel. There were 166 doctors (13 percent of the total) who lived in such inaccessible parts of East Anatolia that it was necessary to mail questionnaires.

Interviewers were mainly recruited from university students in Ankara. Of thirty-two candidates, the sixteen that were chosen had the following backgrounds: two were fourth year and ten were sixth year medical students, two were students from the Academy of Social Science, one was a graduate student in education, and one was a teacher who had previous experience in demographic surveys.

It was calculated that one interviewer could reach sixty-five doctors in a six-week period. Each interviewer received ten days' training which included five days of theoretical instructions, three days of practical interviewing of Ankara doctors not in the sample, and two days for discussing their experiences.

Several control methods were used. When an interviewer completed his questionnaires in one region, he returned to Ankara and was sent to another region. To cross-check, he began work in the new region by reinterviewing one-fifth of the doctors who had been seen by the previous interviewer. For a second control check, a page of the questionnaire was mailed to another one-fifth of the doctors who had already been interviewed and the results were compared. This system of checks showed that one interviewer in the Istanbul area had falsified three complete interviews and a portion of a fourth. Consequently, the sixty-seven interviews which this man had conducted were not included and those individuals were reinterviewed. When a doctor was on a holiday or had moved, he was contacted at his current place of residence. The direct cost of interviewing totaled 27,350 TL ($3,040).

Validation of Survey Data

The major part of the data collection was completed within two months. Table 3–7 shows the disposition of the survey efforts and the fact that 18 percent of the sample were out of the country and only 3 percent were not traced or refused to participate.

TABLE 3–7. COMPARISON OF PLANS AND FINAL RESULTS IN COMPLETING DETAILED QUESTIONNAIRE (1964)

	Original plan	Final results as completed	
		No. of doctors	Percent
Interviews completed	848	822	65.5
Mailed questionnaires	62	166	13.2
Doctors known abroad	93	230	18.3
Doctors unknown	254	14	1.1
Doctors refusing interview	—	10	0.8
Doctors not answering mailed questionnaire	—	15	1.1
Total	1,257	1,257	100.0

In the tables which follow there are sometimes small variations in the total number of doctors who responded. These are caused by the few instances in which a particular question was not answered.

In order to determine whether the sample represented the universe, two comparisons were made: by years of graduation (Table 3–8) and by schools of graduation (Table 3–9). These two statistical checks showed that the doctors in the sample had the same distribution as the doctors in the universe in two major parameters.

TABLE 3–8. COMPARISON OF UNIVERSE AND SAMPLE GROUP BY YEARS OF GRADUATION (1964)

| Years of graduation | % of doctors | | % sample to total |
	Universe (N = 12,472)	Sample (N = 1,257)	
1923–9	3.8	4.2	11.1
1930–9	10.6	11.3	10.8
1940–9	31.8	31.9	10.1
1950–9	39.2	37.3	9.6
1960–3	14.6	15.3	10.6
Total	100.0	100.0	10.1

$x^2 = 3.15$
$.75 > p > .50$

TABLE 3–9. COMPARISON OF UNIVERSE AND SAMPLE GROUP BY SCHOOLS OF GRADUATION (1964)

| Medical schools | % of doctors | | % sample to total |
	Universe (N = 12,472)	Sample (N = 1,257)	
Ankara	20.5	19.2	9.4
Istanbul	76.5	77.8	10.3
Izmir	1.6	1.4	8.6
Foreign	1.4	1.6	11.8
Total	100.0	100.0	10.1

$x^2 = 2.63$
$p > .50$

Even though the response rate was unusually high, similar statistical checks were made to be sure that the respondent group represented the sample. Both comparisons showed good concordance (Tables 3–10 and 3–11).

TABLE 3–10. COMPARISON OF SAMPLE GROUP AND RESPONDENT GROUP
BY MEDICAL SCHOOL (1964)

Medical schools	% of doctors	
	Sample group ($N = 1,257$)	Respondent group ($N = 988$)
Ankara	19.2	18.7
Istanbul	77.8	78.2
Izmir	1.4	1.5
Foreign	1.6	1.6
Total	100.0	100.0

$x^2 = 2.97$
$.75 > p > .50$

TABLE 3–11. COMPARISON OF SAMPLE GROUP AND RESPONDENT GROUP BY SEX
(1964)

Sex	% of doctors	
	Sample group ($N = 1,257$)	Respondent group ($N = 988$)
Male	85.4	86.7
Female	14.6	13.3
Total	100.0	100.0

$x^2 = 100$
$p > .25$

Age and Sex Distribution

The age and sex distribution of the respondents are shown in Table 3–12. The average age of female doctors was 36.5 and of male doctors 41.5 years. The over-all average age was 40.8. The proportion of women doctors in Turkey has been increasing steadily and in recent years has exceeded one-third. This is in accord with a general tendency around the world.

TABLE 3–12. AGE AND SEX DISTRIBUTION OF DOCTORS (1964)

Age groups (years)	Number of doctors		% female to male	Total	
	Male	Female		No. doctors	%
24 or less	8	8	50.0	16	1.6
25–9	87	27	31.0	114	11.5
30–4	135	33	24.4	168	17.0
35–9	188	19	10.1	207	21.0
40–4	161	23	14.3	184	18.6
45–54	202	16	7.9	218	22.1
55–64	74	5	6.8	79	8.0
65 or more	2	—	—	2	0.2
Total	857	131	15.3	988	100.0

The Growing Financial Insecurity of Doctors

Economic considerations are especially significant in under-standing the growing dissatisfaction of Turkish doctors. One indi-cation of their insecurity is the finding that almost a fifth of Turkish doctors have emigrated. When doctors now living in Turkey were asked why their colleagues leave, over two-thirds said that the principal reason was low income.

Doctors' Income

The most direct information on income was obtained from the doctors' census which asked for a straightforward statement of total income. Of the 7,396 doctors responding only 195 or 3 percent said either that they did not know their income or that they received none. The figures included all income from private practice, sal-aries from the Ministry of Health, and other sources. The sur-prising willingness of this many doctors to respond seemed to be partially, at least, because they were eager to register complaints about their income. Among doctors more satisfied with their in-come the response rate was presumably lower and they were prob-ably among the 26 percent nonrespondents. The median monthly income for all doctors of 2,381 TL ($264) is therefore considerably below other estimates.

Another indication of the generally low financial remuneration of doctors is the basic government salary scale. A physician's starting salary is 675 TL/month ($75). Increments are obtained at three-year intervals to a maximum, after thirty years' service, of 2900 TL/month ($322). By comparison, the U.N. estimate is that the average Turkish wage earner received an income of 420 TL per month in 1964 for a six-day week.

Table 3–13 and Figures 3–1 and 3–2 provide a comparison of total incomes and private incomes of general practitioners and specialists and indicate the financial reason for the trend toward specialization. Whereas half of general practitioners earn more than 1,751 TL per month, 76 percent of specialists earn more than this amount. Incomes of specialists are greater than those of general practitioners mainly because the specialists make an average of 711 TL more from private practice (Figure 3–2).

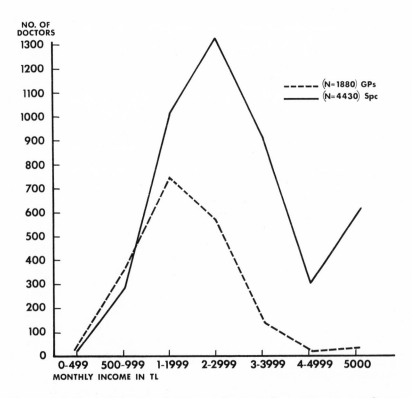

FIGURE 3–1. TOTAL MONTHLY INCOME OF GENERAL PRACTITIONERS AND SPECIALISTS, AS REPORTED IN DOCTORS' CENSUS.

Doctors' Financial Expectations

The doctors in the sample survey were asked to indicate what they considered a reasonable minimum income (Table 3–14). Even though their goals were scarcely exorbitant, the present government salary scale is only one-third to one-fourth as much. As might be anticipated, doctors with foreign experience expected a higher income than those who had remained in Turkey. This information is consistent with the 1963 experience in recruitment for the nationalization plan in eastern Anatolia. The salary was four to five times the government standards and doctors applied in adequate numbers even though the assignments were in primitive rural areas.

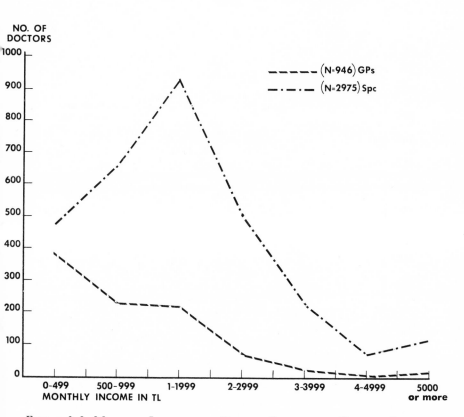

FIGURE 3–2. MONTHLY INCOME FROM PRIVATE PRACTICE OF GENERAL PRACTITIONERS AND SPECIALISTS, AS REPORTED IN DOCTORS' CENSUS.

TABLE 3–13. CUMULATIVE COMPARISONS OF TOTAL MONTHLY INCOME OF GENERAL
PRACTITIONERS AND SPECIALISTS (1964)
FROM CENSUS STUDY

	General practitioners	Specialists	Total	Excess of specialists over general practitioners
Income exceeded by ¾ of doctors (TL)	1,111 ($123)	1,791 ($199)	1,505 ($167)	680 ($75)
Median income (TL)	1,751 ($194)	2,684 ($298)	2,381 ($264)	933 ($103)
Income exceeded by ¼ of doctors (TL)	2,513 ($279)	3,765 ($418)	3,401 ($377)	1,252 ($139)

TABLE 3–14. DOCTORS' STATEMENT ABOUT MINIMUM INCOME CONSIDERED
REASONABLE (1964)
FROM 10% SAMPLE STUDY

Marital status	Minimum mean monthly income
Single doctor	2730 TL = $303
Married doctor without children	3640 TL = $404
Married doctor with 3 children under 16 years of age	4297 TL = $477

Multiple Jobs

In order to earn enough money, many doctors hold two and sometimes three or four different jobs. Each additional job makes it more difficult to do efficient and competent work. The multiple work pattern is summarized in Table 3–15. One half of the doctors have two or more jobs.

Sixty-four percent of doctors who work for the government find it is necessary to have more than one job in order to support their families. Table 3–15 shows that fifty-two of the fifty-eight doctors with three or more jobs were Ministry employees. In fact, the work

TABLE 3–15. NUMBER OF JOBS HELD BY DOCTORS[a] (1964)
FROM 10% SAMPLE STUDY

No. of jobs	Ministry of health doctors		Other doctors		Total	
	No.	%	No.	%	No.	%
One	145	35.8	342	63.3	487	51.5
Two	208	51.5	192	35.6	400	42.3
Three	50	12.2	6	1.1	56	5.9
Four plus	2	0.5	0	0.0	2	0.3

[a] Thirty-nine doctors were not included because they were not practicing and four did not answer this question.

load in Ministry jobs has been kept light with the expectation that outside work will continue as the generally accepted pattern.

The Urban Concentration of Doctors

Almost two-thirds of all doctors in Turkey are located in the three metropolitan areas—Istanbul, Ankara, and Izmir. An additional one-fourth are in smaller cities and only one-eighth are in villages and towns (Table 3–16). The maldistribution of doctors is even more evident when one realizes that only 5 percent of the total population lives in the three big cities where 61 percent of the doctors work. The rural areas where 68 percent of the population lives are served by 13 percent of the doctors.

As expected, proportionately more female than male doctors are located in metropolitan areas. The percentages are seventy-six for women doctors and fifty-nine for men. More graduates of Ankara

TABLE 3–16. DISTRIBUTION OF DOCTORS BY PRESENT PLACE OF RESIDENCE (1964)
FROM 10% SAMPLE STUDY

Place of residence	No. of doctors	% of doctors	Percentage distribution of total population in Turkey
Village and town	132	13.4	68.0
City (provincial center)	249	25.2	26.8
Metropolitan	607	61.4	5.2
Total	988	100.0	100.0

Medical School stayed in metropolitan areas than did Istanbul graduates. This is probably because Ankara, as the newer of the two schools, has been absorbing its graduates into its own hospital and clinic facilities. None of the sixteen Turkish graduates of foreign medical schools in the sample was practicing in a rural area.

A strong association was demonstrated between the doctor's present place of practice and his father's education, which is also an indication of the family's socioeconomic position (Table 3–17). Doctors whose fathers had secondary or university education were more likely to be found in urban areas.

TABLE 3–17. RELATIONSHIP BETWEEN DOCTOR'S PRESENT PLACE OF RESIDENCE AND
HIS FATHER'S EDUCATION (1964)
FROM 10% SAMPLE STUDY

| Present place of residence | Father's education | | |
	None or primary (%)	Secondary or university (%)	Total (%)
Rural	44.7	55.3	100.0
City	36.0	64.0	100.0
Metropolitan	21.1	78.9	100.0
Total	28.1	71.9	100.0

Also related to the family's financial status is the observation that if the doctor had received a medical school scholarship for his living expenses, he was more apt to be practicing in a rural community (Table 3–18).

Doctors were then asked to recommend administrative policy changes which would make rural service more attractive. Three major suggestions were made: 49 percent mentioned better financial remuneration, 24 percent stressed suitable living conditions, and 12 percent emphasized providing necessary professional equipment. It is of interest that these are not in the same order of importance as those listed in the problems of rural service.

From time to time the government has recommended a law that would force doctors to go to rural areas. The fact that only one percent of the sample were in accord indicates that there would be strong opposition from the medical profession.

TABLE 3–18. CORRELATION BETWEEN RECEIPT OF MEDICAL SCHOOL SCHOLARSHIP AND
DOCTOR'S PLACE OF PRACTICE (1964)
FROM 10% SAMPLE STUDY

| | Previous place of practice | | | |
Scholarship	Mostly rural (%)	Mostly city (%)	Mostly metropolitan (%)	Total (%)
Had scholarship (N = 522)	27.4	29.7	42.9	100.0
No scholarship (N = 452)	15.3	20.4	64.4	100.0
Total	21.8	25.3	52.9	100.0

$x^2 = 65.83$
$p > .005$

Distribution of General Practitioners and Specialists

General practitioners were about equally distributed between metropolitan areas and cities and rural areas. However, with 68 percent of the total population living in rural areas the proportionate neglect is obvious. Furthermore, the distribution of specialists was even more biased toward metropolitan areas.

The difference in distribution of general practitioners and specialists is most marked when the location of the doctor during his total period of practice is analyzed. Almost half of general practitioners as compared with only 14 percent of the specialists had previously practiced mainly in rural areas. The percentages for mainly metropolitan practice were 61 percent for specialists as compared with 25 percent for general practitioners (Table 3–19).

Of the doctors who began their professional careers in rural areas, half eventually specialized. Of those who then completed specialty training, 40 percent returned to rural areas. Of the doctors who began their careers as general practitioners in rural areas and never specialized, the vast majority remained there.

Trend Toward Specialization

Only 24 percent of the doctors in the sample were general practitioners. The remaining 76 percent were either specialists (62 percent) or were in specialty training (14 percent). At Turkey's

TABLE 3–19. DISTRIBUTION OF GENERAL PRACTITIONERS AND SPECIALISTS BY
PREVIOUS PLACE OF PRACTICE (1964)
FROM 10% SAMPLE STUDY

Specialty	Previous place of practice			
	% Mostly rural ($N = 214$)	% Mostly city ($N = 250$)	% Mostly metropolitan ($N = 518$)	Total % ($N = 982$)
General practitioner ($N = 235$)	48	27	25	100
Specialist ($N = 747$)	14	25	61	100

present stage of health development there is general agreement that this imbalance is inappropriate. Table 3–20 shows the types of specialization, with about 37 percent of doctors in medical, 28 percent in surgical, and 8 percent in laboratory specialties.

TABLE 3–20. DISTRIBUTION OF DOCTORS BY SPECIALTIES (1964)

Specialty	No. of doctors	Percent
General practitioner	238	24.1
Internal medicine	193	19.6
Neurology and psychiatry	29	2.9
Pediatrics	67	6.8
Medical subspecialties	77	7.8
General surgery	85	8.6
OB-GYN	101	10.2
Surgical subspecialties	96	9.7
Laboratory specialties	84	8.5
Academic specialties	9	0.9
Preventive, judicial, and occupational medicine	'9	0.9
Total	988	100.0

To get subjective evaluation of the need for specialized care, general practitioners were asked what percentage of their patients should have gone to specialists. They said they could adequately handle 75 percent of their patients without referral to specialists for diagnosis or treatment. When the reverse question was posed to the specialists they answered that 40 percent of their patients might have been adequately handled by a skillful general practitioner. If these estimates are valid, then it is apparent that general practitioners could care for more of the present patient load.

Most hospitals in Turkey operate with a small nuclear staff of specialist physicians supplemented by a large number of residents training to be specialists. These residents receive low salaries, thus permitting the hospital to operate on a minimum budget. Administrators have tended to increase the number of residencies beyond their teaching facilities. Academic standards have been kept low so that residents can readily pass the examinations and other requirements for specialization. Present policies need to be changed in two directions. Until the standards are elevated, there is little hope that the present exaggerated trend toward specialization will be reduced. Conversely, it is probable that with a changed emphasis in medical education plus appropriate rewards in terms of prestige, income, living and working conditions, the status of general practitioners can be raised.

Factors Influencing Doctors to Specialize

Most specialists said that the main reason for specializing was the greater prospect of professional success and security. They also felt they would be more useful to society by developing competence in a particular field. Furthermore, they enjoyed the higher prestige attached to specialization. General practitioners naturally had a somewhat different view of the reasons why so many doctors specialize. They felt that specialists were mainly interested in extra income (Table 3–13), better living conditions, and greater prestige.

Only 45 percent of specialists said they felt competent to practice medicine immediately upon graduation while 54 percent of general practitioners answered this question positively. The feeling of inadequacy at the time of graduation was equal for male and female doctors. Almost all of the respondents said that the main reason for lack of confidence was insufficient practical training.

Specialization was more common among doctors whose fathers had more than primary education. Sixty-three percent of doctors whose fathers had little or no education became specialists as compared with 75 percent whose fathers had secondary or university training.

Doctors were asked to rank their impression of public opinion of the relative importance of various medical specialties. Such a ranking is obviously a combination of how doctors *want* the public to feel and what the public *actually thinks* (Table 3–21).

TABLE 3–21. RANK ORDER OF DOCTORS' IMPRESSIONS OF POPULAR ATTITUDES
TOWARD VARIOUS SPECIALTIES (1964)
FROM 10% SAMPLE STUDY

Medical specialty	% considered very important
Surgery	90.1
Internal medicine	88.8
Pediatrics	71.3
OB-GYN	67.6
Radiology	52.4
Ophthalmology	45.6
Psychiatry	16.9
Bacteriology	3.5
Public health	1.8

Though not unexpected, it is of serious national concern that public health was ranked lowest in importance. This has wide implications since it portends a continuing difficulty in recruiting public health specialists for the expanding programs of the Ministry of Health.

Preference for Work in Private Offices or Public Institutions

Of the doctors in the sample, 807 (82 percent) said they preferred to work in public institutions, whereas 171 (17 percent) preferred private offices. Ten did not answer. Of 494 doctors who worked either full time or part time in private offices, 376 (76 percent) said that they would rather work in public institutions if salaries were adequate.

Of 272 doctors whose fathers had either no education or only primary schooling, 22 percent preferred private practice; of 693 doctors whose fathers had secondary or university education, 16 percent preferred private practice. This suggests that doctors who come from a relatively deprived family background are somewhat more inclined to try to better their financial situation through private practice.

Attitude toward Nationalization of Health Services

The overwhelming majority of doctors in the sample approved the plan for nationalization of health services (Table 3–22). Indeed, 69 percent were entirely in accord and 16 percent were at least partly in favor of the plan. This makes a total positive response of 85 percent. Among the 8 percent of doctors who were against the plan, no correlation could be found with factors such as sex, father's education or foreign experience.

TABLE 3–22. ATTITUDES OF TURKISH DOCTORS TOWARD THE GOVERNMENT'S PLAN FOR NATIONALIZATION OF HEALTH SERVICES (1964) FROM 10% SAMPLE STUDY

Attitude	No. of doctors	Percent
In favor	687	69.5
Against	87	8.8
Partly in favor	158	16.0
Have no idea	56	5.7
Total	988	100.0

The 245 doctors who either completely disapproved or were only partly in favor of nationalization of health services were asked to indicate their main objections. Thirty-one felt it might put an end to private practice, 48 said the pay was insufficient, 15 objected to the difficult working conditions, 8 felt that special skills would be lost, and 4 objected to the specified obligatory work period. Almost half of the 158 doctors partly favoring nationalization recommended various modifications such as obtaining additional money from direct contributions from the people, and a few thought that other public services should also be nationalized.

Doctors' attitudes toward nationalization of health services are clearly influenced by the amount of activity in their own practice. Those who saw only a few private patients (less than five patients per day) were more in favor of nationalization than doctors who saw many patients. This association proved to be highly significant statistically (Table 3–23).

Difficulties Encountered by Medical Officers of Health

As in many other countries, Turkish doctors are not attracted to public health as a specialty and they do not have much respect for

TABLE 3–23. ATTITUDES OF DOCTORS TOWARD NATIONALIZATION RELATED TO
NUMBER OF PATIENTS EXAMINED IN PRIVATE OFFICES PER DAY (1964)

Attitude toward nationalization	Number of patients seen per day			
	4 or less (%)	5–14 (%)	15 or more (%)	Total (%)
In favor (N = 325)	65.5	30.7	3.8	100.0
Not in favor (N = 55)	41.8	56.4	1.8	100.0
Total	61.9	34.4	3.7	100.0

$x^2 = 13.71$
$p > 0.005$

its practitioners. One reason why the work of Medical Officers of Health has been unpopular is because they have in the past been essentially the only doctors serving the large numbers of people in rural populations. The experiences of Medical Officers of Health may help define the problems of rural health services and suggest ameliorative proposals which will attract more doctors to rural areas.

Although 362 (37 percent) of the 988 respondents had worked as Medical Officers of Health, only 28 (3 percent) were currently working in this capacity. Of the 362 doctors, 348 were male and 14 were female. They were asked to list the major difficulties which they had faced as Medical Officers of Health. Ministry of Health regulations list 103 duties for the position, but usually no special training is provided. This overload of duties led 31 percent to say that general working conditions were unsatisfactory. About 37 percent said that their worst problem had been to cope with legal responsibilities, such as pronouncing an individual to be under the influence of alcohol or acting as coroner.

Poor provincial administration was mentioned by 13 percent. More specifically, the doctors resented the tendency of the *kaymakam* (government official in charge of the *kaza* or district) to exert authority beyond his technical competence. Most irritating is the rule that Medical Officers of Health must constantly check in and check out with the *kaymakam*. Even if the doctor is going to a rural area as part of his regular work, he must inform the *kay-*

makam. Poor administration by the Ministry of Health was referred to by 4 percent, 3 percent mentioned low income and, surprisingly, only one percent complained about living conditions.

Doctors who had been Medical Officers of Health tended not to specialize, with only 44 percent becoming specialists as compared with 70 percent of other doctors. Doctors who had received scholarships while in medical school were more likely to seek public health positions. More than half of those who had received scholarships worked in public health as compared with one-fifth of the non-scholarship students. The high correlation suggests that financial need is an important factor and recruitment for public health might be helped by more scholarship programs.

Subsidy of Medical Education through Scholarships

Scholarships in Turkey are used mainly for living expenses. The only academic expenditure required from students is a tuition fee of about $10 per year.

Fifty-four percent of the respondents received a scholarship (Table 3-24) for one or more years of their education and 32 percent received a full six-year scholarship. The financial factor is indicated by the finding that doctors who came from families where the father had little or no education had significantly more scholarship support.

TABLE 3-24. DISTRIBUTION OF DOCTORS RECEIVING SCHOLARSHIPS COMPARED WITH FATHERS' EDUCATION (1964) FROM 10% SAMPLE STUDY

	Fathers' education		
Scholarship	None or primary (%)	High or university (%)	Total (%)
Never received (N = 448)	38.8	49.3	46.3
Received (N = 519)	61.2	50.7	53.7
Total	100.0	100.0	100.0

$x^2 = 8.6$
$.01 > p > .001$

The career choice of doctors who had received scholarships suggests a practical means of attracting doctors to rural service. More scholarships and other assistance to rural and financially needy students might increase this trend.

Dynamics of Migration of Doctors to and from Turkey

For many countries a major problem is the "brain-drain" of highly trained technical personnel. Turkish doctors can readily enter the world market for physicians because medical skills and knowledge comprise a "global currency." Turkey has a great investment in each doctor since the government pays most of the costs of medical education. The growing demand for doctors makes this professional leakage particularly serious.

There has been much speculation but little factual data on the magnitude of the loss of Turkish doctors to other countries. Little is known about whether the reasons are professional and personal or whether something in their medical education and professional training promotes interest in working abroad.

Since 230 (18.3 percent) of the 1,257 doctors in the random sample were living abroad, it was estimated by simple extrapolation that a total of 2,248 Turkish doctors were outside the country. Within a 95 percent confidence interval the number of doctors known to be abroad then would be between 2,114 and 2,382. The distribution of doctors overseas by sex and year of graduation and by foreign country is shown in Tables 3–25 and 3–26. By far the greatest proportion are doctors who graduated five to fifteen years ago and who would have completed their military training.

TABLE 3–25. DISTRIBUTION OF TURKISH DOCTORS KNOWN TO BE ABROAD BY SEX
AND YEAR OF GRADUATION (1964)
FROM 10% SAMPLE STUDY

Year of graduation	No. of doctors		Total	
	Male	Female	No.	%
Prior to 1940	13	1	14	6.1
1940–9	55	4	59	25.6
1950–9	117	21	138	60.0
1960–3	12	7	19	8.3
Total	197	33	230	100.0

TABLE 3–26. DISTRIBUTION OF DOCTORS KNOWN TO BE ABROAD BY FOREIGN
COUNTRY (1964)
FROM 10% SAMPLE STUDY

| | No. of Doctors | | Total | |
Country	Male	Female	No.	%
U.S.	53	9	62	27.0
West Germany	74	12	86	37.4
Canada	13	3	16	7.0
Other countries	14	4	18	7.8
Countries unknown	43	5	48	20.8
Total	197	33	230	100.0

West Germany and United States are the two countries attracting
the most Turkish doctors. Extrapolating the sample ratio to the
total population, an estimated 607 Turkish doctors are in the U.S.
and 832 in West Germany.

All doctors in the sample were asked to give their opinions concerning why doctors leave Turkey: 68 percent said that there was
insufficient income; 12 percent mentioned lack of professional
advancement; 6 percent said that professional relationships among
Turkish doctors were poor with intense competition and little
regard for ethics; 6 percent mentioned the more comfortable living
conditions in foreign countries; and 5 percent referred to inefficiency
in health administration. Of the 988 doctors who responded to our
questionnaire, 245 had had professional experience abroad. Of these
245, 118 (48 percent) hoped to go abroad again. Doctors who went
abroad immediately after graduation seemed to have doubts about
their professional competence and felt the need for further training.

Analysis of the duration of the stay abroad for the 75 doctors in
the sample who returned from the U.S. showed that 95 percent
stayed at least a year and over a third stayed more than five years
(Table 3–27). The average length of stay in the U.S. was more than
twice that in Germany, France, England, and Switzerland.

In a special survey which was done as part of this study by Dr.
Donald Ferguson, information was gathered on Turkish doctors
now in the U.S. The American Medical Association has a comprehensive record on IBM cards of all physicians registered for practice
or in regular institutional appointments in the U.S. According to
these records, in 1965, 538 Turkish medical graduates were in the

TABLE 3–27. DURATION OF OVERSEAS EXPERIENCE OF TURKISH DOCTORS*

Experience	Total %
Less than 6 mo.	5.3
1–2 years	38.6
3–4 years	21.3
5–9 years	33.4
10 or more years	1.4

*Seventy-five doctors who had been in U.S.

U.S. (compared with the probably more complete estimate of 607 from the sample survey) and 90 percent were males; 80 percent were graduates of Istanbul and 20 percent of Ankara medical schools. Almost all had graduated at least five years before and 85 percent were graduates from the fifteen-year period between 1945 and 1959. Only one percent were interns; almost 30 percent were residents or fellows in training, and the remainder were in hospital or private practice. Of the more than two-thirds who were not in training, almost half were salaried employees of hospitals, almost 40 percent were in private practice, and the remaining 10 percent were in other activities such as teaching or research. Almost 40 percent were fully licensed which is a clear indication of their intent to remain in the U.S.

Doctors Who Leave the Profession

Rumors periodically circulate that, because of poor income, doctors are leaving medical practice and going into other "businesses." However, of the 988 doctors interviewed, only 39 (3.9 percent) were not currently working as doctors. Twelve of the nonworking doctors were older physicians who had already practiced twenty-five or more years and had retired. If these doctors were excluded, there would be only 27 doctors (2.7 percent) who had stopped professional work. Nine of these 27 doctors (or one-third) were female, but this is still only 6 percent of all female doctors in the sample. Of these 27 doctors all but 6 housewives were engaged in remunerative work: 13 were employed by drug firms either as administrators or as advertising representatives, 4 owned farms, 3 were members of Parliament or the Senate, and 1 doctor was employed as a clerk. Twenty-four doctors gave reasons for stopping professional work: 9 were able to increase their yearly income, 4 said their working conditions had been unsuitable, and

11 left for health and other personal reasons. Included in the latter group were 7 female doctors.

Attitudes toward Recommending a Career in Health Services

When doctors in the sample were asked whether they would encourage their children to enter the same profession, responses were almost evenly split: 468 doctors said they would encourage their children to become doctors and 499 doctors said they would not. Those who were favorable ranked their reasons as follows: (a) because the doctors themselves enjoyed their work, (b) because they liked to help people, (c) because of family tradition and pride, and (d) because the profession has prestige. The negative reasons stressed the inadequate pay and unsuitable working conditions, followed by the long and expensive period of education, and finally the fact that the doctors themselves were not happy in their work and that prestige has been reduced.

These answers were quite different from responses on the possibility of nursing careers; 730 out of 973 doctors (75 percent) said they would *not* encourage their daughters to become nurses. There were no significant differences between the feelings of male and female doctors or specialists and general practitioners. Older doctors were more favorable toward nursing careers than younger doctors. Because nurses have more prestige and better working conditions in most Western countries than in Turkey, it was thought that Turkish doctors who had been abroad would have more positive attitudes. This correlation was highly significant; doctors with foreign experience were more inclined to encourage their daughters in nursing careers. Doctors who had spent most of their professional lives in metropolitan areas were also more favorable.

Negative reasons were as follows: 56 percent felt nursing has little prestige; 12 percent said that the Ministry of Health shows a lack of concern for nursing; 12 percent mentioned difficult working conditions; and 7 percent said that training is inadequate.

THE PRIVATE SECTOR*

Transitional State of Private Medical Practice in Turkey

The difficult transition from a predominantly private to a mixed public and private system dominates present medical care

*Parts of this section are adapted from material prepared by Professor Mark Perlman of the University of Pittsburgh.

developments in Turkey. The forces and trends affecting private practice are still sufficiently strong to require attention in over-all manpower planning.

A preliminary generalization is that the private sector demand for health manpower has been saturated. Doctors are finding it increasingly difficult to get established in private practice. Medical manpower for the public sector will, however, not become automatically available under the present inadequate standards of remuneration and services.

In Turkey, as in many countries, medicine has been a private and highly individualistic profession. Medical practitioners considered independent private practice to be the ultimate professional and ethical norm. As long as medical care was mainly for those who could pay sufficient fees to make medical practice lucrative, there were strong economic incentives to maintain private practice. The shift to public support introduced new economic forces which now apply particularly to young doctors entering practice. Looking ahead, however, as economic conditions in Turkey improve, the proportion of persons able to pay for private care will undoubtedly increase and the private sector may expand gradually.

The rapid growth of the public sector has been built on and mixed with private practice in a most confusing way. In 1876, the government began providing a limited amount of financial support for poor patients who were cared for by private practitioners and this was gradually expanded. In 1923, a law formalized the relationship with private practitioners by stating that any doctor who accepted these subsidies was a government employee. Because of the ready support from government funds, most Turkish practitioners have gradually moved into a mixed medical practice.

Another factor is that many practitioners, especially surgeons, need hospital facilities. Access to such facilities is most readily obtained by appointment in a government hospital. Surgeons often manage to arrange the admission practices so that patients have to be seen first in the specialist's private office. To complete the intricate picture a number of private hospitals are staffed by public sector physicians who hold part-time appointments.

Many doctors start their professional work from the slim security of a government position. They build up progressively the proportion of time spent in private practice after government service hours. Their primary effort is to concentrate on private practice because it is more lucrative. Especially deleterious are the pressures which are placed on patients from the public facility to visit the doctor privately in order to get the best service.

Two sequences may cause practitioners to shift to full-time private practice. First, an occasional practitioner may do so well in private practice that he deliberately chooses to give up his government job. More commonly, the government may routinely transfer the doctor. Because he would lose his private-practice income which is usually greater than his government salary, he often decides to resign. He may eventually secure another government appointment.

Although private practice will undoubtedly continue to develop as an important system of care for urban areas, the needs of rural areas are particularly jeopardized by the present mixed pattern of care. Doctors naturally devote their major time and effort to the activity that provides their main source of income. In addition to all of the intrinsic difficulties which will be discussed in the next section, rural work has little prospect of extra income. Similarly, the chances of attaining the desired comprehensive approach to preventive and curative services are slim until doctors are satisfactorily paid for preventive services.

Also to be considered as a numerically important, though less tangible, part of the total private-practice system is the role of nonmedical practitioners. The great volume of medical care for the rural and the poor is being provided, not by doctors, but by the many indigenous practitioners who are clearly in the private sector. These practitioners attempt to meet the social, psychological, and convenience needs of patients. Their continuing success is an indication of the relative importance of such private sector inducements.

Data on private sector practice are hard to collect because of the natural suspicion of private physicians about the research objectives. In spite of expected defensive attitudes, data were obtained which seem valid even though they are not sufficiently complete to be conclusive. They confirm sound general impressions about private practice and offer some new insights. More important, the gaps in information suggest further studies.

Who Are the Physicians in the Turkish Private Sector?

Basic data on private practitioners were taken from the doctors' census. Almost one-tenth of the 7,273 respondents or 679 physicians classified themselves as being wholly or predominantly in private practice.

The median age of the private sector physicians was 43.8 years, somewhat older than their public sector counterparts who were 38.7 years. This difference is shown in Table 3–28 by both age and length of practice. An obvious explanation is that success in the private sector takes time since reputation of skill is passed mainly by word of mouth.

TABLE 3–28. PERCENTAGE OF PRIVATE AND PUBLIC SECTOR PHYSICIANS IN TURKEY (1964) ACCORDING TO AGE AND LENGTH OF PRACTICE, FROM CENSUS STUDY

	Private sector	Public sector
	(679 physicians) (%)	(6,594 physicians) (%)
Age		
Less than 25 years	0.3	3.1
25–34	15.5	31.9
35–49	62.1	53.5
More than 50	22.1	11.5
Total	100.0	100.0
Length of practice		
Less than 3 years	1.5	7.2
3–10	16.4	29.1
More than 10	82.1	63.7
Total	100.0	100.0

The symmetry of the geographical distribution of physicians in both sectors is contrary to the general impression that the public sector allocates its roster of physicians differently from the spontaneous market control of the private sector (Table 3–29). This means that public sector services have not yet fulfilled one of their main obligations which is to equalize the distribution of personnel according to population ratios.

The specialization pattern of private-sector physicians shows a broad range of activities. Over 35 percent are general practitioners, 37 percent are in medical specialties, 21 percent are in surgical, obstetrical, and gynecological specialties, 6 percent are in laboratory specialties and only 0.1 percent are in occupational and preventive medicine.

TABLE 3–29. PERCENTAGE OF PRIVATE AND PUBLIC SECTOR PHYSICIANS IN TURKEY
(1964) ACCORDING TO LOCATION OF PRACTICE
FROM CENSUS STUDY

Location	Full-time private sector (679 physicians) (%)	Public sector (6,594 physicians) (%)
Istanbul	34.9	30.6
8 large cities	32.8	39.2
16 small cities	16.2	14.3
42 towns and rural areas	16.1	15.9
Total	100.0	100.0

Who Are the Patients?

Numbers

A questionnaire was sent to each of the 679 physicians who classified themselves in the census survey as wholly or predominantly
in private practice. Information was sought on patients who visited
the doctor's office within a one-week period during November,
1964, and 509 doctors responded. The over-all average of thirty-one
patients per week on the basis of a six-day week comes to only
five patients per day (Table 3–30).

The 112 general practitioners reported that they saw an average
of thirty-nine patients per week. There was a general correlation
between number of patients and years in practice (Table 3–30).
The 397 specialists saw fewer patients with no clear correlation
with years in practice. The average was twenty-eight-patient visits
per week. The fact that neither specialists nor general practitioners
are busy probably means that the fewer patients seen by specialists
is due to their higher fees rather than to a deliberate limitation of
patient load in order to spend more time with each patient.

Size of community had no consistent influence on numbers of
patients seen (Table 3–31). If patient load can be used as an in-
dicator of unmet demand, the figures suggest that general practitioners are busiest in the biggest cities and rural areas, whereas
specialists are slightly busier in the smaller towns and rural areas.
This is, of course, the converse of the actual distribution of physicians.

TABLE 3–30. PATIENTS SEEN IN SURVEY WEEK (NOVEMBER, 1964) BY 509
PRIVATE PHYSICIANS ACCORDING TO LENGTH OF TIME IN PRACTICE

	Length of time in practice			
	3 years	3–10 years	10 years+	Total
General practitioners				
No. of physicians	45	19	48	112
Average patient visits per physician	33	38	44	39
Specialists				
No. of physicians	0	83	314	397
Average patient visits per physician	0	25	29	28
Total physicians	45	102	362	509
Average patient visits for total of physicians	33	27	31	31

TABLE 3–31. PATIENTS SEEN IN SURVEY WEEK (NOVEMBER, 1964) BY 509 PRIVATE
PRACTITIONERS ACCORDING TO SIZE OF COMMUNITY

	Istanbul	Cities over 100,000	Cities 50– 100,000	Towns and rural areas 50,000 and under	Total
General practitioners					
No. of physicians	81	24	42	15	112
Average patient visits per physician	40	46	32	42	39
Specialists					
No. of physicians	141	120	112	24	397
Average patient visits per physician	26	30	27	34	28
Total physicians	172	144	154	39	509
Average patient visits for total of physicians	29	33	28	34	31

These figures were strongly corroborated in a separate study. Data on patients seen in private practice were also gathered in the detailed questionnaires sent to a 10 percent random sample of all physicians in Turkey. Out of a total of 988 respondents, 594 said they spent sufficient time in private practice to have a private office or clinic, obviously a larger group than those who participated in the survey week. Almost 90 percent said they saw less than 10 patients per day and two-thirds reported 4 or less per day (Table 3–32). The over-all average was 5.3 patients per day as compared with the average of 5 per day reported during the special survey week.

TABLE 3–32. NUMBER OF PATIENTS SEEN PER DAY IN DOCTORS' PRIVATE OFFICES
OR CLINICS (1964)
FROM 10% SAMPLE STUDY

Number of patients examined	All doctors with private offices		Doctors in full-time private practice	
	No.	%	No.	%
4 or less	310	62.6	52	44.1
5–9	134	27.1	33	27.9
10–14	32	6.5	14	11.9
15–19	110	2.0	4	3.4
20 or more	9	1.8	6	5.1
No answer	—	—	9	7.6
Total	495[a]	100.0	118	100.0
Average patients per day	5.3		7.4	

[a] Ninety-nine additional doctors did not respond.

The numbers of patients seen by the 118 physicians engaged in full-time private practice were separately analyzed (Table 3–32). The average number of patients examined daily was 7.4 which is only two more per day than were seen by all part-time private practitioners.

Neither study gives evidence that Turkish private practitioners are overwhelmed by public demand for their services.

Age Distribution of Patients

A great deal about the patient population going to private physicians can be learned from their age distribution. Since base figures for the number of potential patients in each category are not available, only intergroup comparisons can be made.

Almost 50 percent of the patients seen during the survey week were in the age group of 15–44 and 22 percent were 45–64. The high proportion of visits by patients in the working age group of 15–44 years is contrary to the usual U-shaped curve found in most morbidity and health care surveys. It is clear that wage-earning age groups are in fact receiving most of the private medical care. Figures 3–3 and 3–4 compare the age distribution of private patients seen during the survey week in Istanbul and rural areas. These percentages are calculated on a per-year-of-age group basis

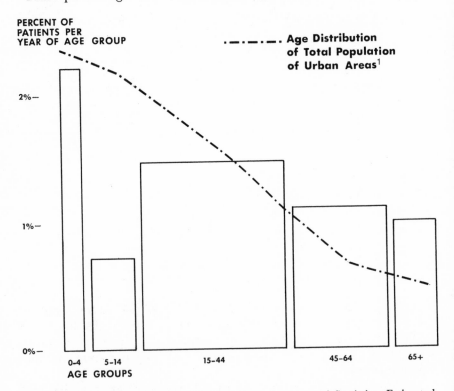

PERCENT OF
PATIENTS PER
YEAR OF AGE GROUP

·—·—·—· Age Distribution
of Total Population
of Urban Areas[1]

2%—

1%—

0%—

0-4   5-14   15-44   45-64   65+

AGE GROUPS

[1] 1960 Population Census of Turkey, State Institute of Statistics. Estimated national totals based on 1 percent sample.

FIGURE 3–3. AGE DISTRIBUTION OF PRIVATE PATIENTS SEEN BY 172 PHYSICIANS IN ISTANBUL DURING SURVEY WEEK, NOVEMBER, 1964 (N = 4861). (TOTAL PERCENT FOR AGE GROUP MAY BE OBTAINED BY MULTIPLYING PER YEAR PERCENT BY NUMBER OF YEARS IN AGE GROUP.)

because of the unequal time span included in age groupings. The marked difference between the age distribution of patients in Istanbul as compared with rural areas is that there were many more older patients and fewer children. Smaller cities and towns showed the expected intermediate age grouping.

Rural-Urban Differences in Patients

In 1963 a nationwide "Population Growth Study" surveyed a random sample of the total population of Turkey. It was financed by the Ministry of Health and the Population Council and the field work was supervised by Dr. George W. Angell and the Test

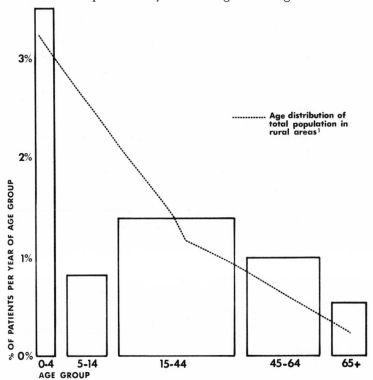

[1] 1960 Population Census of Turkey, State Institute of Statistics. Estimated national total based on 1 percent sample.

FIGURE 3–4. AGE DISTRIBUTION OF PRIVATE PATIENTS SEEN BY 39 PHYSICIANS IN SURVEY WEEK, NOVEMBER, 1964 (N = 5114). (TOTAL PERCENT FOR AGE GROUP MAY BE OBTAINED BY MULTIPLYING PER YEAR PERCENT BY NUMBER OF YEARS IN AGE GROUP.)

Bureau of the Ministry of Education. Demographic data were collected and variables relating to the possibility of starting a national family-planning program were studied. Through the excellent co-operation of those responsible, three questions about morbidity and the sources of medical care were included in this household survey.

Because more than half of the reported utilization of medical services was in the private sector, these data are included in this chapter. Twenty-two percent of rural people and 30 percent of urban people said they had received medical treatment during the previous month in 1963. Table 3–33 shows that less than 50 percent of health facilities used were publicly financed. Rural and urban populations had remarkably similar patterns of utilization except for greater use of indigenous and paramedical personnel in rural areas. Other data reported in a subsequent section suggest that the low figures on utilization of indigenous personnel are probably due to gross under-reporting because this was an official survey and their practice is legally prohibited.

TABLE 3–33. PERCENTAGE DISTRIBUTION OF THE KIND OF HEALTH FACILITIES USED BY INDIVIDUALS REPORTING ILLNESS IN PREVIOUS MONTH IN RURAL AND URBAN SAMPLES
(POPULATION GROWTH STUDY, 1963)

	Residence	
Type of health facilities	Urban (%)	Rural (%)
Public hospital and dispensary	46.1	41.1
Private and semiprivate doctor	40.1	36.4
Pharmacist	7.6	11.4
Other trained health personnel	1.6	3.1
Indigenous health personnel	4.6	8.0
Total	100.0	100.0

In the same survey the time needed to reach different health facilities was recorded (Table 3–34). Public facilities were more readily accessible in urban areas while in rural areas nonmedical personnel were most accessible. Both urban and rural people are apparently willing to devote far more travel time to get help from the private sector than from the public. It was also found that in rural areas most people traveled by foot to see trained health personnel. In urban areas most people used motor vehicles or horses, donkeys, and carts.

TABLE 3–34. PERCENTAGE DISTRIBUTION OF PATIENTS BY TIME NEEDED TO REACH DIFFERENT TYPES OF HEALTH FACILITIES, BY RURAL AND URBAN RESIDENCE (POPULATION STUDY, 1963)

Kind of health facilities	Urban residence				Rural residence			
	Less than 1 hr.	1–3 hrs.	More than 3 hrs.	Total	Less than 1 hr.	1–3 hrs.	More than 3 hrs.	Total
Public hospital and dispensary	61.8	25.8	12.4	100	17.3	31.1	51.6	100
Private and semiprivate	35.4	53.9	10.7	100	11.3	16.5	72.2	100
Pharmacist	50.0	44.7	5.3	100	36.0	45.6	18.4	100
Other trained health personnel	56.2	31.3	12.5	100	38.7	35.5	25.8	100
Indigenous health personnel	58.7	39.1	2.1	100	45.0	35.0	20.0	100
Total	50.1	39.2	10.7	100	20.1	27.9	52.0	100

How Much Do Private Physicians Earn?

As difficult as it is important is the effort to obtain accurate data on private-practice income. Several different approaches have been tried in this study. They all suffer from the expected biases toward under-reporting. The data are included here because they are of interest methodologically and because, whatever their limitations, they provide some previously unavailable information on which judgments can be based and further investigations planned.

The doctors' census questionnaire carried a separate question asking directly for monthly income from private practice. It should be noted that most doctors also derived income from nonprivate sources. Forty-five percent of all doctors reported that they earned less than 1,000 TL ($111) from private practice, and another 30 percent said they earned less than 2,000 TL($222). The median private-practice income for the country as a whole was reported to be 1,193 TL ($134) per month (Table 3–35). Turkey in Europe reported the lowest median income of 981 TL ($109), corroborating other evidence that Istanbul is heavily oversaturated with private practitioners. The Mediterranean and Black Sea coast regions reported the highest median private-practice income of 1,493 TL ($165) and 1,449 TL ($161) respectively. The expected progressive falling off of private-practice income was observed in the eastern part of the country.

TABLE 3–35. MEDIAN MONTHLY INCOME FROM PRIVATE PRACTICE OF GENERAL PRACTITIONERS AND SPECIALISTS ACCORDING TO REGIONS (1964) FROM DOCTORS' CENSUS

Regions	No. of GP	No. of spec.	Ratio of GP to spec.	Median monthly income (TL)		
				GP	Spec.	Total physicians
Turkey in Europe	202	928	0.18	680	1,037	981
Black Sea coast	122	240	0.34	857	1,714	1,449
Marmara and Aegean Sea coasts	200	633	0.24	652	. 1,387	1,201
Mediterranean Sea coast	75	199	0.27	790	1,788	1,493
West Anatolia	53	189	0.22	446	1,476	1,258
Central Anatolia	157	629	0.2	821	1,455	1,293
Southeast Anatolia	49	45	0.52	586	1,848	1,047
East Anatolia	88	112	0.44	490	1,593	986
Total	946	2,975	24.0	693	1,392	1,193

There was a marked economic differential between the private-practice income of general practitioners and specialists (Table 3–35). The median private practice income of all general practitioners was reported as 693 TL ($77) which was only half the income of specialists, 1,392 TL ($155) per month. Part of this income differential may be due to the relatively greater proportion of general practitioners who work in low-income areas. That this is not a sufficient explanation is shown by the fact that Turkey in Europe has the lowest ratio of general practitioners to specialists (.18) but also the lowest median income (Table 3–35).

Four rank-order correlations were done (Table 3–36). First, the rankings by regions of median incomes of general practitioners and specialists were compared. The R calculation came to exactly zero, indicating that there was no relationship between the regions where general practitioners and specialists had high incomes. A significant correlation was found ($R = .83$) between the ratio of numbers of general practitioners to specialists and the regional rank order of specialists' income. This means that specialists' incomes were highest where the supply of specialists was low relative to the number of general practitioners. The general practitioners' income did not show this relationship ($R = -.19$), suggesting that only specialist income depends on the balance of general practitioners to specialists. Also when the differences between the median monthly incomes of specialists and general practitioners were ranked, a significant correlation with the ratio of general practitioners to specialists was found ($R = .83$). Again, this indicates that specialists' incomes were highest relative to general practitioners' incomes precisely in the areas where the specialist ratio was lowest.

TABLE 3–36. REGIONAL RANK-ORDER CORRELATIONS OF RELATIONSHIPS BETWEEN FOUR FACTORS RELATING TO PRIVATE-PRACTICE INCOME OF GENERAL PRACTITIONERS AND SPECIALISTS (1964), FROM DOCTORS' CENSUS

Regions	(A) Income of general practitioners	(B) Income of specialists	(C) Difference between income of specialists and general practitioners	(D) Ratio of numbers of general practitioners to specialists
Turkey in Europe	4	8	8	8
Black Sea coast	1	3	5	3
Marmara and Aegean Sea coasts	5	7	6	5
Mediterranean Sea coast	3	2	4	4
West Anatolia	8	5	3	6
Central Anatolia	2	6	7	7
Southeast Anatolia	6	1	1	1
East Anatolia	7	4	2	2

1. GP's income (A) vs. specialists' income (B) by region $R = 0$.
2. Specialists' income (B) vs. ratio of GP to specialists (D) $R = .83$ (Significant)
3. GP's income (A) vs. ratio of GP to specialists (D) $R = -.19$
4. Differences between incomes of GP's and specialists (C) vs. Ratio of GP's to specialists (D) $R = .83$ (Significant)

The over-all relationships between the incomes of general practitioners and specialists are also shown graphically by regions in Figures 3–5, 3–6, and 3–7. Wide variation in the income distribution of general practitioners is evident. In Central Anatolia and the Black Sea coastal regions the general practitioners appear to be relatively better off than in the other regions. By contrast, the private practice income of specialists shows considerable uniformity in all regions, and this is in spite of the observation noted before that numbers of specialists vary widely from region to region.

These data suggest that spontaneous adjustments lead specialists to limit their numbers in each region so as to maintain a relatively high private-practice income. General practitioners, on the other hand, take care of the practice that is left over and therefore end up with much more regional variation in income.

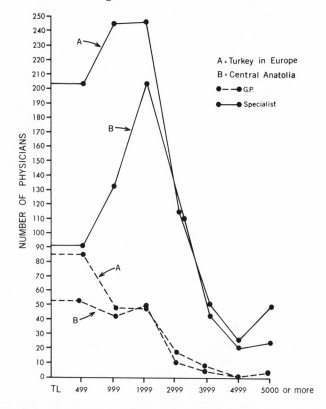

FIGURE 3–5. COMPARISON OF MONTHLY INCOME OF GENERAL PRACTITIONERS AND SPECIALISTS ACCORDING TO REGIONS (FREQUENCY DISTRIBUTION OF NUMBERS OF DOCTORS IN EACH INCOME BRACKET).

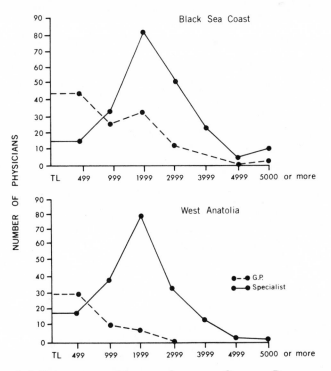

FIGURE 3–6. COMPARISON OF MONTHLY INCOME OF GENERAL PRACTITIONERS AND SPECIALISTS ACCORDING TO REGIONS (FREQUENCY DISTRIBUTION OF NUMBER OF DOCTORS IN EACH INCOME BRACKET).

Average Fees in Private Practice

Throughout this manpower study data have been gathered in several different ways to provide cross-checks. Because of doubts about the validity of data gathered directly from the doctors' census, special efforts were made to develop indirect ways of estimating private-practice income. In the 10 percent sample survey, 509 doctors replied to a question about usual, lowest, and highest fees charged for office visits and 409 responded to a similar question on home visits.

There was a considerable difference in fees charged by general practitioners and specialists in their private offices. About 95 percent of general practitioners said their usual office fee was 20 TL ($2.22) or less. Only 22 percent of specialists were in this category whereas 63 percent said their usual fee was 21–40 TL. Arithmetic means showed that specialists' fees were almost double those of general practitioners (30 TL vs. 16 TL).

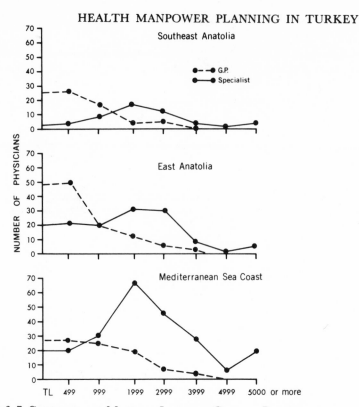

FIGURE 3–7. COMPARISON OF MONTHLY INCOME OF GENERAL PRACTITIONERS AND SPECIALISTS ACCORDING TO REGIONS (FREQUENCY DISTRIBUTION OF NUMBERS OF DOCTORS IN EACH INCOME BRACKET).

Similarly, there was a sharp difference in fees charged for house calls. About 70 percent of general practitioners said they would charge 20 TL or less as a usual fee whereas less than 7 percent of specialists gave this answer. More than half of the specialists charged 21–40 TL, 26 percent charged 41–60 TL, and 13 percent charged more than 60 TL. Average home-visit fees were 20 TL for general practitioners and 39TL for specialists.

Geographical differences were not marked. Fees of general practitioners showed remarkable uniformity in all regions for both office and home visits. Specialists in the larger cities charged higher fees for both office and house visits than in smaller cities. This clear response to the market economy probably occurs because of concentration in the larger cities of both professors and prestigious physicians and also wealthy patients.

The relationships between numbers of patients and fees charged in private offices are summarized in Table 3–37. The uniformity of the general practitioners' fees means that their income is directly related to the number of patients seen, but this has no relationship with the physician/population ratio. Since their fees decrease with the size of cities, specialists have to see more patients in the smaller towns to get more income, and this is related to the specialist/population ratio. The number of specialists diminishes progressively as the cities become smaller.

A further refinement in the sample survey made questioning about income even more indirect. Doctors were asked to estimate the average fees charged by professional colleagues living in the same areas (Table 3–38). There were consistent differences in the

TABLE 3–37. AVERAGE WEEKLY INCOME FROM PRIVATE OFFICE VISITS FROM GP'S AND SPECIALISTS ACCORDING TO POPULATION UNIT (1964) FROM 10% SAMPLE STUDY

		Size of Individual Population Unit			
	Istanbul	Cities with population over 100,000	Cities with population 50,000– 100,000	Cities with population 50,000 and under	Over-all average
General practitioners					
Av. fee	16	16	16	16	16
Av. patients seen	40	46	32	42	39
Av. income per week	640 TL	736 TL	512 TL	672 TL	624
Number of doctors	31	24	42	15	Total 112
Persons per general practitioner	60,712	254,408	183,559	803,830	
Specialists					
Av. Fee	32	30	28	28	30
Av. patients seen	26	30	27	34	28
Av. income per week	832 TL	900 TL	756 TL	952 TL	840
Number of doctors	141	120	112	24	Total 397
Persons per specialist	13,348	50,881	68,835	502,394	

TABLE 3–38. ESTIMATE OF USUAL FEES PER CONSULTATION CHARGED BY PROFESSIONAL
COLLEAGUES LIVING IN THE SAME AREA (1964)
FROM 10% SAMPLE STUDY

	Private office		Patient's home	
Geographical unit	Total no. of respondent physicians	Average fee in TL[a]	Total no. of respondent physicians	Average fee in TL[a]
Istanbul	170	31	173	44
Cities over 100,000	142	30	139	39
Cities 50,000 to 100,000	159	26	157	34
Cities 50,000 and under	44	25	47	29
Total	515	29	516	38

[a] Arithmetic mean calculated using a 15 TL value for the 0–20 TL category since these fees undoubtedly clustered around 20 TL.

direction of their estimating that colleagues' fees were higher than their own.

The average fee for office visits reported by all doctors for their own practice was 25 TL per patient while their estimates of their colleagues' fees averaged 29 TL. For home visits an average fee of 38 TL was estimated for colleagues as compared with 35 TL for themselves. The differences were consistent regardless of size of the community. In general, it is safe to assume that doctors underestimated both their own and their colleagues' fees.

An additional analysis separated out the fees reported by 118 full-time private practitioners. Their usual fees charged were reported as 27.3 TL and eight doctors (7 percent) said they received an average fee of 50 TL or more.

We now have a second way of estimating monthly income from private practice. The average number of private office patients seen per week by general practitioners (39) multiplied by the mean fee charged (16 TL) gives a mean weekly income of 624 TL ($69.33) or 2,785 ($309.44) per month. The same figures for specialists were 28 visits multiplied by the 30 TL mean fee or 840 TL ($93.33) per week and 3,528 TL ($392.00) per month. Even though these indirect estimates are still probably low, they are more than twice the mean monthly income reported in direct answers to the doctors' census question on private practice income.

The Proportion of Free Care

Private sector physicians claim that they devote much time to "free work." Half of all doctors in the 10 percent sample survey said they gave some free care and half of this group said they received no payment from nearly 20 percent of their patients. About one-tenth of all physicians claimed they provided free care for 50 percent of their patients. These are only off-the-cuff judgments, with no specific effort to record data, and are therefore probably inflated. General practitioners saw somewhat more charity patients than specialists. There also seemed to be more free care provided in the smaller cities and rural areas which may be related to the larger number of general practitioners and the lack of public facilities.

SUMMARY

That the private sector furnishes considerable medical service is evident. It is an important element of the Turkish medical system. Ten percent of all doctors are in full-time private practice. The 45 percent who are part-time spend a significant portion of their working hours in private offices or clinics.

The geographical allocation of private-sector physicians followed closely the public-sector distribution. Fewer than anticipated were located in the Istanbul area, indicating that Istanbul's private sector is entrenched and hard to enter. More important in this comparison is the finding that physicians can make an independent income in the smaller cities of Turkey which are not necessarily pecuniarily poor places. Where money is to be made in Turkey there are doctors to meet the demand, especially because public-sector doctors are so poorly paid that they must supplement their incomes.

Private practitioners are not busy. In two different surveys we obtained figures of about 31 patients per week and 5.3 patients per day as estimated average patient load. When doctors were asked a direct question on monthly income from private practice, they reported low figures. Evidence was obtained indirectly by asking doctors to estimate their average fees and these were then multiplied by their reports of average number of patients. These figures were 2.5 to 4 times higher than the direct estimates and probably represent a closer approximation to the truth. Specialists, of course, command larger incomes than general practitioners. Half of all private practitioners claim that they provide some free care to patients who cannot pay.

ATTITUDES OF TURKISH DOCTORS TOWARD RURAL SERVICE

No research was needed to identify the most acute manpower problem of the national health services of Turkey. As in many countries of the world, the gross maldistribution of the medical profession, with an inordinate concentration of doctors in urban areas, constitutes the greatest single administrative problem. It will be virtually impossible to do much about the health care of the 70 percent of the Turkish population who live in villages until there is a continuing mechanism for maintaining professional contact with these people. Even mass programs such as those for controlling malaria and tuberculosis really cannot be implemented without a basic infrastructure of health services. In the national family-planning program it is becoming increasingly evident that the best way of reaching rural people is through a total network of organized health services, particularly those concentrating on maternal and child health care.

After the law for the nationalization of health services was passed in 1961, a prolonged period of careful preparatory work led to a phased plan of implementation. The province of Mus in eastern Anatolia was selected for the pilot study which began in 1963. Progressive expansion of the total nationalization plan was then started, gradually extending province-by-province from eastern Anatolia toward the west.

The greatest uncertainty in setting up such rural services is the fact that doctors generally do not like to work in rural areas. They have many good reasons for not working in villages. Most health administrators have impressionistic stereotyped explanations for the unfavorable attitudes toward rural work. Although these opinions may have validity for particular situations and times, it is increasingly evident that the problem is too complex to be solved by simplistic answers.

A special study was designed to probe into the balance of factors that influence doctor's attitudes toward rural service. The specific aims of this study were: (1) to improve the methodology of research on professional attitudes; (2) to define the characteristics of doctors willing to accept work in rural areas and to determine how they differ from doctors working in urban situations; (3) to discover the major problems faced by doctors working in rural health centers so that ameliorative measures can be taken by the government; (4) to define the changes that occur during the process of rural adaptation by retesting a group of doctors after they had spent a year working in rural health centers; (5) to gain insight for improving educational programs.

Materials and Methods

Battery of Tests

Of great assistance in planning this research project was a study in India conducted by the Johns Hopkins Division of International Health, on the rural orientation of doctors going through their rural internship. A battery of tests to measure rural attitudes had been developed which included a comprehensive set of questionnaires and a special set of projection tests including a Rural Thematic Apperception Test* (RTAT) and a story completion test. The pictures in the RTAT depict doctors in a variety of village situations. Those taking the test write short stories suggested to them by each picture. A comprehensive coding manual was developed and validated to permit numerical scoring of the stories for the inadvertent and subtle expressions of attitudes, which reveal basic values more reliably than questionnaire responses. Individuals may give the answers that they think are expected on a questionnaire: the projection tests tend to take a biopsy of their deeper feelings.

The battery of tests from India was readily adapted to Turkish conditions. The total battery was administered in a one-hour sitting. New pictures were drawn putting villagers into Turkish clothes and changing village conditions to resemble everyday life in Anatolia. The story completion test was also modified to put the episodes in a Turkish context. The coding manual was rewritten taking examples from stories actually written in Turkey during the pretesting and pilot stages. Since the scoring of projection tests requires special training, two Turkish women were prepared for the work, one a psychiatrist and the other a college graduate.† Both of these women scored each story independently and then reconciled their differences.

*Developed with the co-operation of Dr. David McClelland, Dr. David Winter, and Dr. George Litwin of the Department of Social Psychology, Harvard University.

†Dr. Gulseren Gunce and Mrs. Ustun Kosefoglu.

Sample Selection and Administration of Tests

A two-phase study was done. The first was a cross-sectional sample of four groups of doctors with different exposure to rural service:

1. Recent graduates—doctors who had joined the nationalized health services immediately after graduation and had worked in rural health centers less than five months. There were fifty-eight doctors in this group.

2. Nationalized health service doctors—doctors who had worked in the nationalized health services in Mus Province for more than one year. There were eighteen health unit doctors who could be reached in this group. Their previous experience before joining the nationalized plan was not taken into account because of the intensive recent experience in Mus.

3. Rural practitioners—a group of forty-five doctors who had worked in nationalized health services for less than five months but had practiced previously in rural areas either privately or in government dispensaries.

4. Hospital residents—a control group of forty doctors who had specialty training right after graduation and were working as residents in Ankara hospitals.

When this study started in the summer of 1964, steady recruitment of doctors for the six eastern Anatolia provinces was progressing. The flow of new doctors through the brief orientation process in Ankara was paced at a rate which permitted testing by one staff member. Another staff member went to Mus to test health center doctors there. The Ankara doctors were tested in their respective hospitals.

The second phase of the study was carried out a year later. The Group 1 doctors who had joined the nationalized health services immediately after graduation were retested to get before-and-after responses from the same individuals.

All doctors were assured that their responses would be kept confidential. The uniform pattern of administration was that all tests were given to individuals or small groups by a Turkish doctor on the project staff.

The tests and questionnaires included the following:

1. Demographic data fact sheet: requiring data such as name, address, marital status, educational background, etc.

2. Questionnaire: Covering opinions of doctors about medical specialties, medical training, salaries, and factors that affected their selection of profession.

3. Questionnaire: Including four groups of questions about favorable and unfavorable aspects of work in the nationalization areas, work in health units, and their opinions of villages and villagers.

4. RTAT: Persons taking this test were given thirty seconds to look at a test picture and then were to write in five minutes a story suggested by the picture. Two printed forms, *A* and *B*, were prepared, each with a set of four pictures which produced essentially the same scores for the values scored. The two sets were given alternately in sequence within each group. Care was taken to ensure that if a doctor in Group 1 received Form B the first time, a year later he was given Form A.

5. Story completion test: Four incomplete stories dealing with dilemmas involving hard choices about ethical or rural problems were prepared and pretested. The situations were more structured than the RTAT pictures. The test involved writing the last part of the story to resolve the dilemma or make an appropriate decision.

6. Questionnaire: more questions about the doctor's past and family history, the educational background of his parents and wife (or husband).

The data from the 211 individual tests were hand-tabulated. The numbers were too small to warrant extensive cross-tabulation. Questionnaire responses were recorded on a four-point scale. Since scalar nonparametric data of this kind have no fixed quantitative values, the points on the scale were assigned arbitrary units. The arithmetic means of these arbitrary units scored for each of the items in a question were then placed in rank order. This rather simple rank-ordering of the averaged opinions of each group of doctors provided a ready means for straightforward statistical analysis.

Findings

Demographic Data on the Four Groups of Doctors

1. Age and sex distribution—The average age of the doctors was 26.6 years for Group 1, 32.2 for Group 2, 33.7 for Group 3, and 26.5 for Group 4. It is evident that the eighteen doctors who had been in Mus for a year were mostly older physicians, similar to those in Group 3, who had previously worked in rural areas. Both of these older groups were almost entirely male while more than a third of Groups 1 and 4 were female.

2. Marital status—The percentage of married doctors was 27.6 in Group 1, 88.8 in Group 2, 75.5 in Group 3, and 17.5 in Group 4.
3. Rural-Urban background—Among the 121 doctors working in nationalized health services there were 11 (9.1 percent) with a rural background and among the 40 residents there were four (10 percent).

Professional Preferences

Differences in personal preference for medical specialties (Table 3–39) presumably reflect basic attitudes toward medical work. Public health is surprisingly ranked high by the older doctors in Groups 2 and 3 who had rural experience. General practice is ranked third or fourth by all groups except the hospital residents who ranked it eighth. Pediatrics and internal medicine were the most popular specialties.

TABLE 3–39. DOCTORS' PREFERENCE FOR MEDICAL SPECIALTIES

| | Rank order of preference | | | |
| | Health unit doctors | | | |
Medical specialties (Group No.)	Recent graduates (1)	Nationaliza-tion service doctors (2)	Rural practi-tioners (3)	Hospital residents (4)
1. General practice	3	4	4	8
2. Internal medicine	1	3	2	2
3. OB-GYN	6	7	7	5
4. Pathology (clinical)	11	12	12	7
5. Ophthalmology	9	9	9	10
6. Pediatrics	2	1	1	1
7. Preclinical sciences	11	11	11	12
8. Hygiene and preven-tive medicine (in medical school)	8	6	6	8
9. Psychiatry	7	8	8	4
10. Public health (service)	5	1	2	5
11. Radiology	10	10	10	10
12. Surgery	4	5	5	3

Preferences for various types of professional work varied widely (Table 3–40). Being a health unit physician in a rural area was ranked first by the two groups of older doctors (Groups 2 and 3). The new graduates (Group 1) who were going to rural areas for the first time gave priority to specialty private practice. The hospital residents who probably included graduates with high academic standing in their medical school classes, preferred careers in medical education and research. An interesting finding was that the doctors with the longest experience in rural areas (Group 3) expressed as great an interest in research as the hospital residents.

TABLE 3–40. TYPES OF PROFESSIONAL SERVICE MOST ATTRACTIVE TO DOCTORS

	Rank order of preference			
	Health unit doctors			
Types of work (Group No.)	Recent graduates (1)	Nationaliza- tion service doctors (2)	Rural practi- tioners (3)	Hospital residents (4)
1. Administrative health services, hospital services	8	4	6	6
2. State hospital physician	3	1	4	4
3. General private practice in an urban area	9	6	7	9
4. General private practice in a rural area	7	5	2	8
5. Private hospital physician	2	9	10	5
6. Research	6	7	3	3
7. Military doctor	10	9	9	10
8. Health unit physician in a rural area	4	1	1	7
9. Specialist (private)	1	3	5	2
10. Faculty member at a medical school	5	8	8	1

Evaluation of Preparation for Service

The doctors evaluated their own preparation for various types of medical practice, using as a basis for comparison the standard they would expect in their colleagues. The sharp differences between health unit doctors and residents appear to depend mainly on what the individual actually expected to do. The health unit doctors reflected a realistic acceptance of their future by ranking themselves as best prepared to be health unit doctors and rural general practitioners. The residents felt best prepared for specialty practice and faculty positions.

Another question probed more specifically for the doctor's evaluation of his own competence in specific professional activities. The results showed less clear-cut differentiation of health center doctors from residents (Table 3–41). All groups ranked themselves highest in establishing good relations with patients and their families and most were confident of their ability to treat patients. All groups ranked themselves low in understanding ecological factors in disease causation, in studying health problems, and in obtaining public co-operation on health matters. The residents had more confidence in their general clinical ability and their ability to diagnose diseases. The health center doctors ranked themselves higher in administration and supervision of health units.

Factors Influencing a Career Choice

Surprising uniformity was found in the ranking of factors influencing career choice. All professed high humanitarian and patriotic motivations. Intellectual satisfaction was also important to all groups. Opinions of members of the doctor's family, being near home, and specific working hours had little influence on career selection.

Financial Expectations

Doctors were asked to estimate what they expected as net monthly income ten years from the date of the survey. Residents expected 2100 TL, health unit doctors in Group 1 expected 2400 TL, Group 2 expected 2800 TL, and Group 3 expected 2900 TL as average monthly income. These figures suggest that "monthly income" was misunderstood as monthly salary and merely reflect the differences in years of service of the various groups. Since health unit doctors are not allowed to have private practice, the estimates of monthly income are a fairly realistic representation of present government salary scales.

TABLE 3–41. DOCTORS' OPINIONS ABOUT THEIR PROFESSIONAL COMPETENCE IN
SPECIFIC TASKS REQUIRED IN MEDICAL AND HEALTH SERVICES

	Rank order of competence			
	Health unit doctors			
Medical services (Group no.)	Recent graduates (1)	Nationali- zation serv- ice doctors (2)	Rural practi- tioners (3)	Hospital residents (4)
1. General ability as a doctor	11	11	10	3
2. Diagnosing diseases with simple clinical methods	10	9	12	5
3. Diagnosing diseases by using results of complicated lab. tests	14	15	15	7
4. Understanding environmental, epidemiological and ecologi- cal factors in disease causation	12	13	13	10
5. Treatment of patients	3	5	2	2
6. Establishing good relations with patients and their families	1	1	1	1
7. Dealing with social and emo- tional problems of patients and their families	2	2	5	5
8. Teaching patients practical methods of disease prevention	5	6	2	4
9. Community health education	9	12	9	12
10. Studying health problems and doing research	15	13	14	13
11. Administration and super- vision of health units	8	2	5	15
12. Co-operating with auxiliary health personnel	6	4	7	14
13. Considering the financial situa- tion of the family before deciding on medical care	3	6	4	9
14. Arranging treatment with limited resources	7	8	7	8
15. Obtaining public co-operation on health matters	13	9	11	10

Factors Favoring the Choice of a Career as a Health Unit Doctor

Doctors were asked to rank the factors which would favorably influence them to choose health unit work as a career. All groups agreed in ranking first altruistic motivations, such as helping people in need and serving communities with humanitarian feelings. Factors such as "to have the administrative responsibility of health unit and staff" and "to be an important person in village" or "to meet interesting emergency cases" were ranked low.

Minor differences between health unit doctors and hospital residents were that "combining preventive and curative services" and "organizing health services for a large group of people" seemed somewhat more important to health unit doctors, and "medical care" was ranked higher by the residents. The rural practitioners (Group 3) ranked "having independent control of one's own work program" as second while it was ranked sixth and eighth by Groups 1 and 2, and fourth by the hospital residents.

Negative Influences on the Choice of a Health Center Career

There was remarkable similarity in the rank order of factors which were unfavorable to the choice of rural work. Most important were: "inadequate medicine and supplies," "unqualified assistant personnel," "inadequate transportation and postal services," and "lack of library and research facilities" (Table 3–42). These are tremendously important to responsible administrators because they provide a ranking of what changes need to be made. The uniformity of response is in itself an indication of the strength of agreement among these professional groups.

Differences in ranking between residents and health unit doctors occurred in only a few items. The first was "lack of professional meetings" which seemed important to health unit doctors, whereas "supervision by nonprofessional persons (*kaymakam*, etc.)" was ranked high by residents and doctors just completing a full year's work in a health unit. The two older groups of doctors understandably ranked lack of educational facilities for their children as an important negative factor.

The Work of Health Center Physicians

All groups agreed that tracing the sources of communicable diseases, doing health surveys in villages, taking care of patients, and holding staff meetings with unit personnel to review work done and plan future work should be the main functions of health unit doctors (Table 3–43). However, residents and health unit doctors did not agree on other functions. Residents said that conducting normal deliveries, doing minor surgical operations, setting simple fractures, and personally administering intravenous injections should be included in the regular work of health unit doctors. But health unit doctors did not think that these were as important as some non-clinical functions, such as studying the social structure and factions in villages and personally visiting homes to encourage villagers to build sanitary toilets and improve their water supply. The ninth and tenth items in Table 3–43 are of particular interest. The choice was posed sharply to see whether Turkish doctors might be willing to use auxiliaries for simple curative responsibilities. The uniformity of the conviction that doctors must see all patients must be taken into account in planning new auxiliary programs.

Doctors' opinions of village people were obtained by having them score on a four-point scale a carefully selected set of twenty-five opposite characteristics such as "clean-dirty," "honest-dishonest." All groups of doctors held remarkably similar stereotypes. All considered villagers to be uninformed, patient, introvert, dependent, undernourished, religious, superstitious, and dirty. At the opposite end of the scale they were thought to be friendly, simple, hospitable, appreciative, wise, and generous.

Results of RTAT Projection Test

The Rural Thematic Apperception Test (RTAT) was scored by content analysis for ten different values. Among these values were somewhat intangible qualities, such as, idealism, materialism, personal concern for patients, and scientific concern. Others were more specific in that they reflected both favorable and unfavorable attitudes toward village people or toward medical colleagues and consultants.

To be noted first is the "no score" column because a high score here is indicative of a general lack of interest in the subject and the test. It is not surprising that the hospital residents scored 25 percent whereas the doctors who had just finished a year in the rural areas scored 12 percent, with the other two groups in between (Table 3–44).

All groups scored high in enthusiasm and idealism. The doctors in Group 1 showed the interesting phenomenon of scoring highest in both favorable and unfavorable attitudes toward villagers and village life. These doctors are those who were going to work in nationalization areas right after graduation and apparently the group contained individuals who were still sorting out their feelings about villages. Doctors in Groups 3 and 4 had the least favorable opinions about village life.

TABLE 3–42. RANK ORDER OF FACTORS HAVING UNFAVORABLE INFLUENCE ON
DOCTORS' ATTITUDES TOWARD RURAL HEALTH UNITS

Factors (Group No.)	Recent graduates (1)	Nationalization service doctors (2)	Rural practitioners (3)	Hospital residents (4)
1. Interference with plans for specialization	11	17	22	16
2. Problems maintaining personal cleanliness and grooming of clothes	16	11	17	19
3. Lack of proper housing	6	8	10	8
4. No chance for professional advancement	9	14	20	7
5. Inadequate instruments and equipment	6	14	11	8
6. Objections of wife, husband, or fiance	25	21	25	24
7. Objections of other family members	27	27	27	27
8. Inadequate health unit buildings	11	11	12	16
9. Lack of professional meetings and stimulating professional contacts	2	6	7	13
10. Inadequate transportation and postal services	5	2	5	4
11. Inadequate medicine and supplies	1	4	3	1
12. Lack of library research facilities	2	9	2	4
13. Insufficient social life and lack of recreational opportunities	23	23	18	22
14. Insufficient income	20	22	15	11
15. Unqualified assistant staff	4	3	1	3
16. Lack of variety in clinical work	14	11	18	18
17. Lack of educational facilities for doctor's children	15	4	4	11
18. Lack of experienced specialist consultation for clinical problems	10	9	8	6

Rank order of importance — Health unit doctor

TABLE 3–42 (*continued*)

Factors (Group No.)	Health unit doctor			
	Recent graduates (1)	Nationali-zation serv-ice doctors (2)	Rural practi-tioners (3)	Hospital residents (4)
19. Health hazards for doctor's family	11	7	9	15
20. Supervision by nonprofessional persons (*kaymakam, nahiye muduru, muhtar*, etc.)	8	1	5	2
21. Too many patients	26	25	24	26
22. Fear of losing clinical skills	17	17	21	23
23. Too few patients	19	26	23	25
24. Fear of personal safety	24	23	26	21
25. Political interference	22	16	16	14
26. Difficulties created by medico-legal cases	17	19	13	8
27. Personal problems of living in village	21	20	13	19

Doctors who scored highest in public health interest were in Group 2. This may have been a direct result of the special emphasis on public health in the nationalization plan. Recent graduates in Groups 1 and 4 had the lowest public health scores.

Personal concern for the patient was low in all groups. The highest scientific medical concern was interestingly in doctors in Group 2, who had one year of experience in nationalization areas. As with public health, this may be a reflection of their greater exposure to in-service training.

The highest score for materialistic motivation was in the hospital residents, followed by the more recent graduates among the health unit doctors. There seemed to be no distinct differences between groups in attitudes toward medical colleagues and consultants (D+, D−, and C) except that the doctors who had been in the nationalization program scored slightly higher than the others in their favorable attitudes toward medical colleagues.

TABLE 3–43. FUNCTIONS EXPECTED OF HEALTH UNIT DOCTORS

	Rank order of importance			
	Health unit doctors			
Functions (Group No.)	Recent graduates (1)	Nationali- zation serv- ice doctors (3)	Rural practi- tioners (3)	Hospital residents (4)
1. To conduct normal deliveries	19	23	19	5
2. To conduct complicated deliveries	23	21	24	22
3. To check statistical data col- lected by assistants on births, deaths, and illnesses and to write official reports	5	12	8	5
4. To do health surveys in villages	3	6	3	4
5. To study the social structure and factions in villages and the beliefs of villagers	8	9	8	19
6. To do emergency surgical operations	20	19	21	16
7. To attend meetings of "com- mittee of elders," *kaymakams,* and *nahiye mudurus* as necessary	22	19	18	20
8. To do minor surgical operations and set simple fractures	12	9	10	3
9. When the number of patients exceeds 100, to see only criti- cal patients and arrange for patients with simple condi- tions such as cold and diarrhea to be seen by a nurse or *saglik memuru*	25	25	26	26
10. To see each patient person- ally even if 100 patients or more come to the unit every morning	7	6	6	7
11. To administer personally all intravenous injections	20	22	22	12
12. To trace sources of communica- ble diseases and arrange control measures	1	2	1	2
13. To arrange group meetings for health education	14	15	15	10

TABLE 3–43. (*continued*)

Functions (Group No.)	Rank order of importance			
	Health unit doctors			
	Recent graduates (1)	Nationali- zation serv- ice doctors (2)	Rural practi- tioners (3)	Hospital residents (4)
14. To take care of patients staying in the health unit	3	2	3	1
15. To give instruction on pre- vention to patients attending the unit	15	6	12	14
16. To supervise family planning and maternal and child health polyclinics (out-patient)	18	16	13	21
17. To do home visits personally and encourage villagers to build sanitary toilets and water systems	9	14	13	18
18. To check the work-schedule of public health nurses, midwives, and *saglik memurus*	2	1	2	9
19. To work in the field with as- sistant personnel each week	11	2	6	16
20. To do school health examina- tions	9	9	10	10
21. To hold staff meetings to review work done and plan future work	6	5	5	7
22. To make the laboratory tests if there is no technician in the unit	16	12	15	14
23. To increase the number of patients coming to the poly- clinics by giving only one or two days' medication	26	26	25	25
24. To administer intramuscular injections	24	24	23	24
25. To do daily administrative work, and from time to time write reports	16	17	17	23
26. To visit patients at home, when necessary, without pay	13	17	20	12

TABLE 3–44. SCORING OF RTAT STORIES FROM FOUR GROUPS OF TURKISH DOCTORS

Groups	No. of respondents	No. of stories	Number of scores[a]										
			E	V+	V−	PH	P	Sc	M	D+	D−	C	No score
Recent graduates (1)	58	232	48 (21)	52 (22)	66 (28)	39 (17)	8 (3)	18 (8)	15 (6)	33 (14)	24 (10)	24 (10)	42 (18)
Nat. service doctors (2)	18	72	12 (17)	15 (21)	14 (19)	20 (27)	1 (1)	10 (14)	3 (4)	15 (21)	10 (14)	7 (10)	9 (12)
Rural pract. (3)	45	180	41 (23)	26 (14)	46 (25)	37 (21)	6 (3)	10 (6)	8 (4)	23 (13)	24 (13)	16 (9)	35 (19)
Hospital residents (4)	40	160	30 (19)	24 (15)	36 (22)	25 (15)	5 (3)	11 (7)	13 (8)	21 (13)	14 (9)	12 (7)	40 (25)

[a]Figures in parentheses in these columns show the percentage of stories reflecting a specific value.

E   = Enthusiastic and/or idealistic
V+ = Favorable reference to villagers and village life
V− = Unfavorable reference to villagers and village life
PH = Reference to public health
P   = Personal concern for patient
Sc = Scientific medical concern

P-Sc = Both P and Sc are present
M   = Materialistic concern
D+ = Favorable mention of the behavior of a medical person
D− = Unfavorable mention of competence or behavior of a medical person
C   = Need for consultation

Results of Uncompleted Stories

The one-paragraph stories concerned either ethical problems faced by doctors or specific choices relating to rural service. There were four such stories which were scored according to a coding manual similar to that used for the RTAT scoring (Table 3–45). The highest "no scores" were again in Group 4 followed closely by Group 1. Even more than in the RTAT, Group 3 scored highest on enthusiasm and idealism. On the other hand, the highest N+ (favorable reference to nationalization of health services program) was in Group 2, who had just completed one year of experience in the nationalization area. A markedly low N+ coinciding with a high N− (unfavorable reference to nationalization program) was found in the hospital residents. The highest Sp (desire to specialize) was understandably in the hospital residents.

The highest PH (public health emphasis) was in Groups 2 and 3. This confirms the influence of rural experience in helping doctors understand the importance of public health. The attitudes toward village life did not conform precisely to RTAT findings, but were more consistent in that reciprocal shifts between V+ and V− were observed. Groups 2 and 3, with the greatest village experience, had the most favorable attitudes toward village life. Differences in "materialistic concern" were not marked but Group 3, who were the oldest, showed the greatest concern.

Comparison of Results in Two Tests of Recent Medical Graduates after an Interval of One Year

In August, 1965, one year after the original tests, a project physician visited eastern Anatolia to reinterview the Group 1 doctors who had joined the nationalized health services shortly after graduation. Of the original fifty-eight doctors, five were doing their compulsory military service. Two female doctors had left to work in urban areas. Of the remaining fifty-one doctors, only one refused to be reinterviewed. (The rank-order numbering of the first interview in this series is somewhat different from the rank orders of Group 1 in the previous section because the total number was reduced from fifty-eight to fifty.)

Specialty Preference and Career Choice

Personal preference for medical specialties changed slightly during the year. Obstetrics and gynecology moved from sixth to third and pediatrics moved from second to first place. General practice declined in rank order from third to fifth place.

TABLE 3–45. SCORING OF UNCOMPLETED STORIES FROM FOUR GROUPS OF TURKISH DOCTORS

Groups	No. of respondents	No. of stories	Number of scores[a]								
			E	N+	N−	PH	V+	V−	Sp	M	No score
Recent graduates (1)	58	232	46 (20)	89 (38)	28 (12)	37 (16)	22 (9)	16 (7)	19 (8)	29 (12)	30 (13)
Nat. Service doctors (2)	18	72	9 (13)	35 (49)	1 (1)	16 (22)	12 (17)	2 (3)	— (—)	10 (14)	3 (4)
Rural pract. (3)	45	180	45 (25)	75 (42)	17 (9)	40 (22)	25 (14)	12 (7)	18 (10)	32 (18)	11 (6)
Hospital residents (4)	40	160	21 (13)	43 (27)	33 (21)	24 (15)	13 (8)	16 (10)	24 (15)	19 (12)	23 (14)

[a] Figures in parentheses in these columns show the percentage of stories reflecting a specific value.

E = Enthusiastic and/or idealistic
N+ = Positive attitude toward nationalized health services
N− = Negative attitude toward nationalized health services
PH = Reference to public health or preventive emphasis
V+ = Favorable reference to villagers or village life
V− = Unfavorable reference to villagers or village life
Sp = Desire to specialize
M = Materialistic concern

The most marked change in rank order of factors influencing career choice was the sharp decline in the influence of faculty members, which dropped from third to eighth place (Table 3–46). A slight upward shift occurred in the importance of job security, intellectual satisfaction, and financial income.

TABLE 3–46. CHANGE IN RANK-ORDER OF FACTORS INFLUENCING THE CAREER CHOICE OF PHYSICIANS FOLLOWING A YEAR IN A RURAL HEALTH UNIT

Factors	First interview	Second interview
1. National needs	2	2
2. Opinions of mother, father, wife, husband, or close relatives	9	9
3. To be near home	10	12
4. Prestige	7	7
5. Intellectual satisfaction	4	3
6. Influence of faculty members	3	8
7. Financial income	6	5
8. Job security	5	3
9. Certain working hours	11	10
10. Possibility for free time	12	11
11. Humanitarian feelings	1	1
12. Job openings	7	6

Doctors' Evaluation of Their Own Preparation

The changes that occurred in the doctors' estimates of their formal preparation for specific types of work are hard to explain since they do not seem logically related to their experience. Following a year in a rural health unit, the ranking of their preparation for private specialty practice moved from ninth to first place. This may be these doctors' way of saying that their medical education had really only prepared them for specialty private practice and therefore may perhaps be a criticism of the relevance of their formal preparation. A somewhat smaller shift in the same direction was noted with research and medical school teaching. Conversely, their ranking of their preparation for general practice and administrative services declined sharply—which would fit the interpretation that they had found they were not prepared to do what their present duties demanded.

The one year's rural experience sharply improved the doctors' estimates of their own ability to co-operate with auxiliary health personnel, take responsibility for clinical treatment, and administer health units. They were more aware, however, of their limitations in teaching patients practical methods of prevention, community health education, and providing treatment with limited resources.

Financial Expectations

After a year's work in rural areas these health unit doctors had merely added the normal annual increment to the regular salary allowed by the government. This seems to indicate that they expected to continue in government service.

Attractiveness of Rural Health Service

In order to attract doctors to work in rural areas, it is necessary to clearly define the favorable and unfavorable factors influencing such decisions. The shifts in attitudes as a result of experience in rural health centers are particularly revealing because some marked changes occurred. The favorable factors are shown first (Table 3–47). The factors which moved up in rank order most markedly are concerned with independence and assumption of responsibility for the whole community. "Combining preventive and curative medicine," however, declined sharply. The decline in "contributing to the health needs of the country" shows a more realistic appraisal of the range of their influence.

There were also some significant shifts among the factors unfavorably influencing career decisions about rural work (Table 3–48). Most dramatic was "supervision by non-professional persons (kaymakam, etc.)" which moved from the rank order of eighth to three-way tie for first place along with "lack of professional meetings and stimulating professional contacts" and "inadequate medicine and supplies." Also ranked as more important were "health hazards for the family" and "inadequate buildings and transportation." Moving down to a lower rank were "lack of proper housing" and "inadequate instruments and equipment." It is of interest that the direction of these shifts in general coincided with the attitudes of Group 2 or the doctors who had previously responded after a year in the nationalization plan.

Functions of Health Unit Doctors

Opinions about the role of health unit doctors did not change significantly. Of most interest was a real increase in sense of respon-

TABLE 3–47. CHANGE IN FACTORS HAVING FAVORABLE INFLUENCES ON
DOCTORS' ATTITUDES TOWARD RURAL WORK AFTER A YEAR'S SERVICE IN A
RURAL HEALTH UNIT

Factors	First interview	Second interview
1. Combining preventive and curative medicine	1	5
2. Helping people in need	3	3
3. Meeting interesting emergency cases	10	9
4. Contributing to the health needs of the country	4	8
5. Having administrative responsibility for health unit and staff	11	11
6. Organizing health services for a large group of people	6	6
7. Studying the community as a whole	8	6
8. Community service with humanitarian feelings	2	1
9. Having independent control of one's own work program	5	3
10. Having independent responsibility for diagnosis and treatment	6	2
11. To be an important person in village	12	12
12. Medical care	9	10

sibility for the doctor's role in relation to auxiliary staff. "Check-ing the work schedules of public health nurses, midwives, and *saglik memurus*" moved from second to first and "staff meetings and field work" also moved up. Some preventive activities became more important, such as "health studies in villages," whereas "tracing sources of communicable diseases and arranging control measures" became slightly less important. Most interesting was the sharp fall in rank order of certain clinical activities, especially minor surgery and setting fractures.

Opinions about village people changed only slightly. Of the twenty-five characteristics scored, the only changes were that doc-tors now considered villagers to be somewhat more careful, patient, and adaptable and less gossipy than before. These indicate a general improvement in attitude toward villagers.

Results of Projection Tests

After a year of rural experience doctors showed far less response to the test than before (Table 3–49). The "no score" figure went up from 18 to 27 percent. There was a sharp decrease in both positive and negative comments about village people. Less dramatic drops occurred in "personal concern for patients" and "material concern." These changes presumably reflect the development of a more casual and realistic attitude toward village work.

TABLE 3–48. CHANGE IN RANK-ORDER OF FACTORS HAVING AN UNFAVORABLE INFLUENCE ON DOCTORS' ATTITUDES AS A RESULT OF A YEAR IN A RURAL HEALTH UNIT

Factors	First interview	Second interview
1. Interference with plans for specialization	13	12
2. Problems maintaining personal cleanliness and grooming of clothes	16	19
3. Lack of proper housing	6	13
4. No chance for professional advancement	9	10
5. Inadequate instruments and equipment	5	11
6. Objections of wife, husband, or fiance	25	25
7. Objections of other family members	27	26
8. Inadequate health unit buildings	12	9
9. Lack of professional meetings and stimulating professional contacts	3	1
10. Inadequate transportation and postal services	6	4
11. Inadequate medicine and supplies	1	1
12. Lack of library and research facilities	2	7
13. Insufficient social life and lack of recreational opportunities	23	21
14. Insufficient income	18	19
15. Unqualified assistant staff	3	5
16. Lack of variety in clinical work	14	14
17. Lack of educational facilities for doctors' children	15	15
18. Lack of an experienced specialist consultation for clinical problems	10	8
19. Health hazards for doctors' family	11	5
20. Supervision by nonprofessional persons (*kaymakam, nahiye muduru, muktar*, etc.)	8	1
21. Too many patients	26	26
22. Fear of losing clinical skills	20	17
23. Too few patients	18	23
24. Fear of personal safety	24	24
25. Political interference	22	22
26. Difficulties created by medicolegal cases	17	18
27. Personal problems of living in a village	20	16

TABLE 3–49. CHANGES IN THE SCORING OF RTAT STORIES BY TURKISH DOCTORS AFTER ONE YEAR IN A RURAL HEALTH UNIT

	No. of respondents	No. of stories	Number of scores[a]										
			E	V+	V−	PH	P	Sc	M	D+	D−	C	No score
First interview	50	200	30 (15)	49 (25)	55 (28)	38 (19)	5 (2)	13 (6)	14 (7)	28 (14)	22 (11)	21 (10)	35 (18)
Second interview	50	200	35 (18)	9 (4)	24 (12)	32 (16)	— (—)	5 (2)	3 (1)	21 (10)	14 (7)	26 (13)	54 (27)

[a]Figures in parentheses show the percentage of stories reflecting a specific value.

E = Enthusiastic and/or idealistic
V+ = Favorable reference to villagers and village life
V− = Unfavorable reference to villagers and village life
PH = Reference to public health
P = Personal concern for patient
Sc = Scientific medical concern
M = Materialistic concern
D+ = Favorable mention of the behavior of a medical person
D− = Unfavorable mention of the behavior of a medical person
C = Need for consultation

SUMMARY

A detailed analysis of doctors' attitudes toward rural service was carried out with a special battery of questionnaires and projection tests. Comparative data were collected from three groups of doctors with distinctly different backgrounds who were working in rural health centers and from a fourth, or control group, of hospital residents. On one of these groups a one-year followup was also done.

All doctors in rural service differed from the control group in their greater interest in general practice, public health, rural work, and village people. A distinct shift in these directions also occurred during the year of rural service.

The respondents were very frank about what they consider to be the main problems of rural work. Ranking highest as unfavorable factors in both the cross-sectional and longitudinal studies were "inadequate medicine and supplies," "supervision by non-professional persons," "lack of professional meetings and stimulating professional contacts," "unqualified assistant staff," and for the two older groups of doctors, "lack of educational facilities for doctors' children." This listing out of twenty-seven alternatives provides a clear indication of priorities which can be used by government officials in remedying the major obstacles to effective service and recruitment.

Doctors also ranked the importance of health center functions and the relevance of their educational preparation for these functions. It is apparent that the present medical education is not providing doctors with the preparation they need. The health unit doctors stressed the need for them to serve as leaders of the health team with their greatest responsibility being to work with the health unit staff. There was also considerable spontaneous emphasis on the importance of preventive services and community studies.

The greatest strength of the nationalization program is the service motivation of the doctors being attracted to it. Their attitudes reflect altruistic and humanitarian feelings with an awareness of community needs. It is mainly their preparation and the official supporting services that need to be improved.

A CRISIS IN MEDICAL EDUCATION

As important as any other factor in determining the future pattern of health services in Turkey will be the influence of the medical schools. To meet the new and rapidly increasing demands for health

care there will have to be a major reorientation of medical education. Special preparation will be needed to produce the type of doctor required by the new plan for nationalization of health services.
As the leader of the health team, the doctor will be primarily responsible for the quality and quantity of service in the new health centers, as well as in the base hospitals. The doctor will, of course, not
be able to work effectively unless a whole concatenation of changes
is made simultaneously. There must be basic reorganization of the
regional administration and rapid expansion and appropriate utilization of all categories of auxiliaries. Financing of health services
must be expanded within the range of economic reality. Effort
must also be focused on solving the population problem. Central
to all of these innovations is the deliberate and planned production
of a new type of doctor.

The crisis in medical education is one of inner orientation in the
medical schools. The changes needed are more qualitative than
quantitative. It has been said that it is as hard to move a medical
school as it is to move a cemetery. Medical educators are traditionally conservative. They bear a heavy responsibility in preserving
the medical subculture of society. As with any group responsible
for maintaining a long-established set of standards, it is almost reflexive for them to view as a threat any move to change medical
education.

The basic point that needs to be generally recognized by medical
educators is that the best quality of doctor required by the Turkish
health services of the future is not what has been accepted as the
best quality of doctor in Western countries. The patterns of medical care which evolved spontaneously in the affluent economies of
the West were devoted to scientific excellence in diagnostic and
therapeutic facilities. Specialists with the most advanced technical
competence were sought out by patients willing to pay whatever
was necessary to get the best individual care. The resulting sharp
trend toward specialization has developed also because doctors
function most comfortably when they do not have to cover the
whole range of medical knowledge.

As in many developing countries, Turkey's new orientation in
medical services requires that a reasonable and feasible quality of
care be provided for most of the people rather than a highly advanced quality of care for a limited and select group.

After a brief discussion of the history of medical education and the methodology of this study, this chapter presents some descriptive data on the staffing of Turkish medical schools, the present curricula, the administrative organization, and an impressionistic and subjective description of the present methodology of teaching. Attention is then given to three areas which are particularly relevant to the quantitative prospects of increasing the supply of medical manpower without building new medical schools. First, the subject of medical school dropouts is analyzed as an obvious way of increasing the number of graduates with minimal investment. Second, the possibility of reducing the related loss of many extra years as the result of high failure rates in examinations is discussed. Third, the relevance of the prolonged periods now being spent in postgraduate education by so many doctors is questioned. Finally, there is a brief statement of some objectives which need to be built into the new pattern of medical education.

History of Medical Education in Turkey

Medical education began in Turkey more than 700 years ago during Seljuk times. The first systematically organized teaching institution was the Giyasiye Medical School which was established in 1205 in affiliation with the Princess Gevher Nesibe Hospital in Kayseri. Teaching was in Turkish and the medical classics of the famed scientist Avicenna (Ibn Sina) and other writers from Central Asia were translated and used as basic texts. Clinical and theoretical subjects were also included in the medical teaching of Husnu Efendi, a Persian refugee, who was the senior physician at a large two-storied hospital founded in Bursa in the late fourteenth century. Turkey was one of the first countries to use practical bedside teaching. The great medical center founded by Sultan Mehmet II at Istanbul in 1470, which was attached to the first Turkish university, was based on a hospital. Fifteen years later, Sultan Beyazid II opened a large hospital and medical school on the banks of the Tunca River in Edirne. One of the most famous teaching hospitals of ancient times was founded by Emperor Suleiman at Istanbul in 1555. By the seventeenth century most of these institutions had declined in importance. A Western-oriented military medical school was opened in Istanbul in 1827 during the reign of Sultan Mahmut II. Karl Ambrose Bernard of Vienna introduced Western techniques and a new educational program including the use of cadavers for anatomical studies. In 1865 Turkish doctors started a civilian medical school in Istanbul with lectures in Turkish. In 1909 the civilian and military medical schools merged to form the Faculty of Medicine of the University of Istanbul. In a major reorganization in 1932 many German professors were given clinical and laboratory appointments. Even today, the basic pattern of medical education in Turkey continues to show the original strong German influence.

In spite of large classes, the Istanbul Medical School was not meeting the demand for doctors for the whole country. The Ankara University Medical School was established in 1945 and ten years later the Ege University Medical School was opened in Izmir. More recently the Hacettepe Medical School was started, also in Ankara, with the specific objective of experimenting with new educational approaches.

Administration of Medical Schools

A law passed by Parliament in 1946 made the universities autonomous centers of higher learning and research under the Ministry of Education. Each university is administered by an Executive Council headed by the dean. Administrative policy is determined by a Council of Professors who elect a new dean of the Executive Council every two years.

Annual fees of $11 per person are paid by students for registration, training, examinations, and diplomas. Essentially all other financial support is provided by the government.

Student Admission into Medical Schools

For admission to medical school a lycee graduate must take a special entrance examination. In 1964 a unified examination system was accepted by all medical schools with standardized objective tests prepared and conducted by the Test and Measurement Bureau of the Ministry of Education. Applicants are from all over Turkey and the results provide a single pool for selection. Fourteen percent of the students in Turkish medical schools are from foreign countries, mainly the Middle East. Some basic information on the size of the four medical schools is presented in Table 3–50.

Duration of Medical Education and Comparison of Curricula

Medical education takes a minimum of six years, with one year premedical, two years preclinical, and three years clinical work. The school year varies from six to eight months. Oral examinations

TABLE 3–50. BASIC INFORMATION ON FOUR MEDICAL SCHOOLS IN TURKEY (1964)

Medical school	Year founded	Teaching staff[a]	No. of students		Graduates		Annual tuition fees (TL)
			Total enrollment	Admitted in 1963	Turkish	Foreign	
Tip Fakultesi Ankara Universitesi (School of Medicine Ankara University) Ankara	1945	388	1,045	225	80	4	100
Tip Fakultesi Istanbul Universitesi (School of Medicine Istanbul University) Istanbul	1827	553	3,143	636	209	65	100
Tip Fakultesi Ege Universitesi (School of Medicine Aegean University) Izmir	1955	204	568	131	73	3	45.50
Hacettepe Tip Fakultesi Ankara Universitesi (Hacettepe School of Medicine, Ankara University) Ankara	1963	277	100	100	—	—	—

[a]Resident doctors are included.

are given twice a year; they are administered individually and require several additional weeks. In case of failure, a student is allowed to repeat an examination as many as four times.

The curriculum structure is rather traditional and largely theoretical in the three older schools but the new Hacettepe Medical School is experimenting with integrated teaching centered around subjects rather than academic disciplines. In the older schools the premedical year includes approximately equal hours allocated to chemistry, physics, botany, and zoology. In the two preclinical years anatomy, histology, physiology, and biochemistry with some biometry or mathematics are offered. The clinical years include separate courses and exams in the usual subjects, such as microbiology, parasitology, pathology, and pharmacology. Legal medicine, the history of medicine, and medical ethics receive separate attention. Somewhat less than half of the time in the three years is allocated to clinical medicine with separate courses in the four major areas of internal medicine, surgery, obstetrics and gynecology, and pediatrics. In addition, there are ten minor clinical courses in the subspecialties.

Because of its special relevance in developing countries, the teaching of preventive medicine and public health in Turkish medical schools was compared with schools in Iran, Pakistan, and Lebanon. Among the Turkish medical schools, Ankara devotes the greatest number of curriculum hours to preventive medicine and public health. However, the medical schools of Iran and Lebanon are far ahead of Ankara, with Beirut offering an additional three weeks of field study in public health (Table 3–51).

Student–Staff Ratios

A low student-staff ratio is usually considered to be an indication of good quality teaching. What is really important, of course, is the amount of small group contact with teachers to provide discussion opportunities and practical supervision. Detailed data were gathered from the records on the student-staff ratios by course in the three medical schools but they are not presented here because they were still considered inadequate. The student numbers could not be clearly prorated to teaching time because of differences in the balance of large group didactic teaching and small group activities. Attempts to categorize teachers into full time and part time were not meaningful because the really important question is the time they devote to teaching. A full-time faculty member

TABLE 3–51. COMPARISON OF THE TOTAL TIME (HOURS) DEVOTED TO TEACHING PREVENTIVE MEDICINE AND PUBLIC HEALTH IN THE MEDICAL SCHOOLS OF TURKEY, IRAN, PAKISTAN, AND BEIRUT (AMERICAN UNIVERSITY)

Subject	Medical schools of Turkey			Medical schools of Iran		Pakistan	Medical school of Beirut American University
	Ankara	Istanbul	Izmir	Teheran Univ.	Shiraz		
Public health and preventive medicine	160	128	151	224	320	75	292 (and three-week field study)
Epidemiology	32	—	—	32	—	—	—
Biometry	—	60	—	16	32	—	—
Total	192	188	151	272	352	75	292

primarily interested in research or the seclusion of an operating room may spend less time with students than a part-time teacher with an active private practice.

Some over-all comparisons are of interest. The student-staff ratio (including both full-time and part-time teachers) was forty-seven in Istanbul, thirty-seven in Ankara, and nineteen in Izmir. This reflects mainly the size of classes. The staffing of departments seems to be more uniform than class size, especially in basic science departments. In clinical departments the needs of the wards over-shadow teaching requirements. There are always more teachers wanting to participate in clinical teaching and this is reflected in the generally lower student-staff ratios in the clinical subjects.

The Medical Student Dropout Problem and Prolongation of Education

The simplest and most direct measure for increasing the supply of doctors is to eliminate unnecessary waste in the educational sequence. The two obvious major problems are a significant drop-out of medical students and extension of the period of study beyond the prescribed period.

The quantitation of medical student dropouts proved difficult and time-consuming. In early 1964, a statistical clerk went to Ankara and Istanbul medical schools to obtain lists of all registered *entering* students from 1947 to 1956. Similar information on the much fewer admissions to Izmir from 1955 to 1956 was gathered through correspondence. A name-by-name comparison was then made with lists of medical school graduates up to 1964 to record their dates of graduation. This tedious analysis proved to be the only way of calculating the numbers and percentages of medical student dropouts and the numbers of students requiring more than six years to complete the course.

Medical students who had transferred from one school to another were particularly difficult to trace. Students originally registered in Istanbul Medical School who had transferred to Ankara numbered 155 while 83 had transferred from Ankara to Istanbul. This total of 238 constituted 3 percent of all admissions.

A total of 7,006 students matriculated at Turkish medical schools between 1947 and 1956 and 3,912 graduated up to 1964 (Table 3–52). This means that only 55.7 percent graduated and the phenomenal dropout rate is 44.3 percent of all admissions. More-over, the number of registered students who graduated in the prescribed six years was only 1,657 or 23.7 percent. In other words,

TABLE 3–52. NUMBER OF STUDENTS ADMITTED TO THE FIRST YEAR IN ALL MEDICAL SCHOOLS, 1947–56, AND NUMBER OF GRADUATES FROM AMONG THEM, BY YEARS SPENT IN MEDICAL SCHOOL

Medical school	No. of students admitted to 1st yr.		No. of students graduated (in years)										Total no. of graduates	
			6		7		8		9		10 or more			
	No.	%	No.	%	No.	%	No.	%	No.	%	No.	%		%
Ankara	2,127	100.0	581	27.3	301	14.3	164	7.7	81	3.8	101	4.7	1,228	57.8
Istanbul	4,701	100.0	957	20.4	747	15.9	326	6.9	201	4.3	300	6.4	2,531	53.9
Izmir	178	100.0	119	66.8	12	6.7	7	3.9	7	3.9	8	4.5	153	85.8
Grand total	7,006	100.0	1,657	23.7	1,060	15.1	497	7.0	289	4.1	409	5.8	3,912	55.7

32 percent of admissions or 58 percent of the graduated students required *more than six years* to complete their studies. Of these, 6 percent of admissions and 10 percent of graduates required more than ten years to graduate. The over-all average age of medical school graduates was twenty-six years.

The graduation rate in the prescribed six years was 27 percent at Ankara Medical School and 20 percent at Istanbul. The eventual dropout rate was 42 percent at Ankara and 46 percent at Istanbul. Ege Medical School in Izmir, on the other hand, in its short span of operation graduated 67 percent of its registrants in six years and had a dropout rate of only 14 percent.

These findings dramatically point up one of the most serious problems in Turkish medical education. More studies are needed to determine whether these difficulties arise from: inadequate premedical preparation, students' uncertainty about career goals, poor selection of students and a deliberate effort by the faculty to use a high failure rate as a screening process, marriage and child-bearing among female medical students, need for more economic support of students (even though the government is already more liberal than in most countries), poor teaching or inappropriate curriculum, or the wrong kind and excessively high standards of examination. Some medical educators seem to consider a high failure rate to be a status symbol which is equated with high academic standards. Clear demonstrations are needed of ways in which this obvious waste of medical manpower can be corrected.

Postgraduate Training of Doctors

Postgraduate training in Turkey is almost exclusively limited to residency training leading to specialization in one of fifty-eight branches. The almost complete lack of postgraduate short courses makes it nearly impossible for practicing physicians to keep abreast of new developments and to receive continuing intellectual stimulation. There are few medical meetings and minimal access to current literature. Even in daily work there are few opportunities for learning through professional contacts.

The different specialties in which certification is possible have been grouped as follows:
(a) clinical specialties, subdivided into thirty-two branches;
(b) laboratory specialties, subdivided into five branches;
(c) academic specialties, subdivided into six branches;
(d) preventive medicine specialties, subdivided into fifteen branches.

The Ministry of Health maintains a list of public and private hospitals and health institutions where a doctor can receive residency training to become a specialist. In 1964, there were 114 hospitals or health institutions where residents were trained. Although residencies may be both salaried and unsalaried, only 10 percent fall into the latter category. Specialty training is organized by the Ministry of Health, the medical schools, the social insurance institutions, the state economic enterprises, and philanthropic organizations.

Residencies range from two to seven years. Almost all of this time is spent in practical training with limited theoretical teaching. While this balance is basically desirable, it is overdone because of the general problem of residents being used by the hospitals as cheap labor. Little attention has been given to making the period of residency a truly educational experience.

Residents are required to take specialty examinations within a month after completing their training. Between the years 1923 and 1963 there were 7,789 specialty certificates registered by the Ministry of Health, which is 61.5 percent of the total Turkish graduates in those years.

The School of Public Health in Ankara was the first school in Turkey to offer postgraduate training in public health and preventive medicine. The Rockefeller Foundation provided funds for the building, which was completed in 1936, and also some of the first staff members. After being discontinued in 1940 because of the war, teaching was resumed in 1947 with short courses for doctors and paramedical personnel of the Ministry of Health.

In 1958 the School of Public Health was reorganized under the directorship of Dr. Nusret H. Fisek and Diploma in Public Health (D.P.H.) training was started. The two-year program has theoretical courses in the first year and practical training in the second. Only doctors are admitted. The School also conducts annual short-term supplementary courses for Ministry of Health doctors. There are also special training programs in connection with the particular needs of national programs, such as tuberculosis control, or at times of special concern, such as the possibility in 1966 that cholera might spread to Turkey. Auxiliary training programs are conducted in special disciplines such as sanitation and statistics. Other institutions which offer preventive medicine specialty training to doctors are the departments of preventive and community medicine in medical schools, the Central Institute of Hygiene, and Gulhane Military Medical School in Ankara.

Cost of Medical Education

The cost of medical education has, so far, received almost no study in Turkey. In manpower planning, decisions about priorities should include an understanding of cost/benefit implications. Projections of the numbers and functional roles of each category of health worker should take into account the cost per graduate. Of equal interest are the cost implications of maximizing the output of limited educational facilities by increasing enrollment and reducing dropouts.

In Turkey, medical education is financed almost entirely by the central government. There tends to be a high degree of stability with budgets based on previous income. Istanbul Medical Faculty obtains about 95 percent of its income from the central government and Ankara and Ege Medical Schools get about 98 percent.[2] Most of the educational costs come directly from the Ministry of Education, whereas most of the hospital costs are provided by the Ministry of Health.

There are differing views as to what items should properly be included in the costs of medical education. In many countries, it is logical to include private expenditures on education and some measure of earnings foregone by students. In this study both these items were excluded. Private expenditures are less than 3 percent of total expenditures for medical education and are relatively inelastic. Earnings foregone were similarly considered too small to be significant at present levels of unemployment.

The government naturally requires regular budgeting and accounting of subsidized expenditure with uniform financial reports. Such documents as the *Official Annual Budgets* for the years 1954 through 1964 contained valuable information about funds allocated to medical schools. However, these data were not complete enough for a detailed cost analysis. Questionnaires were prepared* to obtain detailed financial data from each medical school for each academic year from 1954 to 1964. A breakdown of funds by categories such as personnel, maintenance, student subsidies, and capital expenses was provided by officials of both medical faculties at Ankara and those in Istanbul and Izmir.

*This study was done by Mr. James Lancaster while on an OECD fellowship in Ankara during the year 1964–5.

Comparison of funds allocated to the medical faculties in the *Official Annual Budgets* and the questionnaire reports of actual expenditures showed major differences in the following items:

1. Istanbul and Izmir medical schools show very few hospital expenses on their budget. Their teaching hospitals have separate budgets and are supported by sources such as the Ministry of Health, municipalities, local authorities, and trustees. These medical schools pay not more than one-fifth of the total expenses of these hospitals. However, Ankara and Hacettepe medical schools pay the total expenses of their hospitals. They benefit only minimally from other hospitals for training purposes.

2. Total annual maintenance and replacement expenditures of those medical schools, which have no hospitals of their own, are also limited in comparison with the medical schools which have assumed direct and complete responsibility for their teaching hospitals.

3. Capital expenditures for Istanbul and Izmir medical schools are shown in the budget of the Ministry of Public Works. Because of the special status of Hacettepe Medical School, capital expenditures are part of its own budget, thus distorting its cost ratios during the years of rapid construction of facilities.

4. New equipment is not considered part of capital investment but is shown as current expenditure in the budget, which makes current cost higher for new medical schools.

The data on annual allocations and expenditures provided by the questionnaire must therefore be accepted with caution because it proved impossible to correct for the major differences in accounting practices. These figures should not be used for comparisons between medical schools, but only as indications of over-all trends. Table 3–53 shows that allocations usually exceeded expenditures by significant amounts.

The increase in total current expenditure in all medical schools in the decade 1954–64 has been so rapid that costs have essentially tripled from about 6 to 20 million TL at Istanbul, 4 to 17 million at Ankara, and 5 to 12 million at Ege (Figure 3–8). A major part of these costs is for manpower.

For planning purposes it is necessary to calculate costs per student. The simplest but least precise method is to simply divide the total annual expenditure by the number of students in a year.

TABLE 3–53. AVERAGE ANNUAL ALLOCATION AS COMPARED WITH AVERAGE ANNUAL EXPENDITURES OF TURKISH MEDICAL SCHOOLS FROM 1954 TO 1964
(TL IN MILLIONS)

| | Ankara | | Istanbul | | Ege | | Hacettepe | |
| | Average annual | | Average annual | | Average annual | | 1964 only | |
	Allocation	Expenditure	Allocation	Expenditure	Allocation	Expenditure	Allocation	Expenditure
Current:								
Personnel	9.13	6.11	9.84	8.04	6.10	5.25	7.81	4.08
Maintenance & replacement	1.64	2.49	0.82	0.74	1.93	1.32	2.96	2.73
In-Hospital training	0.21	0.83	4.40	3.69	2.24	2.21	7.58	0.76
Subsidies	3.90	0.59	0.76	0.02	—	0.04	0.03	—
Total current	14.88	10.01	15.82	13.06	10.27	8.82	18.39	7.57
Capital:								
Investment in buildings		2.55		0.89		0.29	4.47	2.40
Durable goods		0.52		0.44		0.01	1.18	2.46
Total capital	2.46	3.07	1.59	1.33	1.02	0.30	5.65	4.86
Total expenditures	17.34	13.08	17.41	14.39	11.29	9.12	24.04	12.43

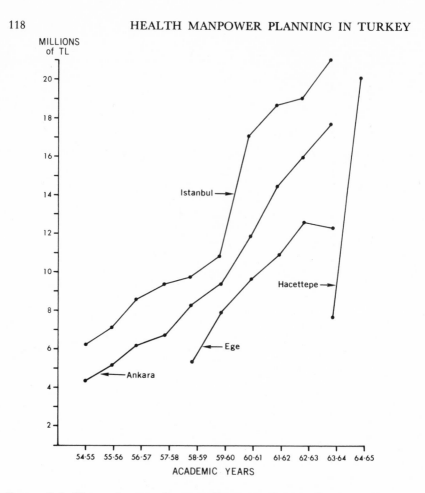

FIGURE 3–8. TOTAL ANNUAL CURRENT EXPENDITURES FOR TURKISH MEDICAL
SCHOOLS (1954–1965).

This method has several limitations:

1. It gives an apparent advantage in low cost per student to
   schools having the largest number of students without regard
   to quality of education or nonmonetary considerations in
   teaching.
2. It also gives an apparent advantage to schools which have a
   high dropout rate and markedly prolonged educational
   intervals, since these students count fully while actually
   representing a lower teaching load and fewer graduates.

According to this calculation in 1954–5 the cost per student was 5,010 TL at Ankara, and 2,522 TL at Istanbul Medical School. In both schools the yearly cost per student was three times this much by 1963–4. Average annual costs per student were calculated for the periods 1954–8, 1958–62, and 1962–4. Table 3–54* relates these costs to enrollment to show that the size of the student body is the important determinant of the major cost differences between schools. Because of the differences in accounting practices outlined above, it must be stressed that variations between schools are more apparent than real. More important are the time trends and the total figures for all medical schools.

Similar calculations can be made using only current expenditures rather than total expenditures as the numerator, thus eliminating the variable capital costs figures. For 1963–4 these costs per student per year are: Ankara, 16,322 TL; Istanbul, 6,549 TL; Ege, 20,477 TL; with an average for all schools of 10,441 TL. Hacettepe was not included in the above tabulations because they do not yet have their full quota of students.

An even more useful estimate of the cost of medical education is obtained by calculating the cost per graduate. This calculation includes in the denominator only the number of students who graduate, and in the numerator the expenditures are expanded to cover the period normally required to complete the course. The primary advantage is that the dropouts and repeaters so common in Turkey are accounted for in the cost. This calculation must be increased first by dividing the average annual cost per student (10,838 TL) by 56 percent which is the percentage of students who ultimately graduate. The average annual cost per graduate then is 19,353 TL. A weighted average of the extra years spent in medical school gives 7.15 years as the average years required to graduate. When these figures are multiplied the average cost of producing a doctor is calculated to be 138,373 TL ($15,374).

The first Five-Year Development Plan proposes five more medical faculties to be started by the Ministry of Health. These schools are to be located in Erzurum, Diyarbakir, Bursa, Sivas, and Adana. The proposal is to admit 50 to 100 students to each class. Construction plans include 400-bed hospitals in Adana and Diyarbakir and 200-bed maternity hospitals in Bursa and Erzurum. With the

*Since Table 3–54 includes capital costs, Hacettepe with its exceptional capital circumstances has been excluded.

TABLE 3–54. AVERAGE ANNUAL ENROLLMENT, TOTAL EXPENDITURE (INCLUDING CAPITAL COSTS), AND COST PER STUDENT BY MEDICAL SCHOOLS BY PERIODS: 1954–8, 1958–62, 1962–4

Medical school	1954–8			1958–62			1962–4		
	Average enroll-ment	Average expendi-ture	Average cost per student	Average enroll-ment	Average expendi-ture	Average cost per student	Average enroll-ment	Average expendi-ture	Average cost per student
Ankara	1,248	8,934,181	7,159	1,019	14,703,453	14,429	1,080	18,155,836	17,183
Istanbul	2,755	9,011,038	3,270	3,088	15,424,392	4,995	3,184	21,343,037	6,703
Ege	—	—	—	598	8,528,310	14,261	602	13,240,687	21,994
Total	4,003	17,945,219	4,482 ($498)	4,705	38,656,155	8,215 ($912)	4,866	52,739,560	10,838 ($1,204)

Source: Questionnaire

exception of the medical school at Erzurum which is to begin taking students in 1966, these faculties cannot start functioning before 1968 and will not graduate a class until after 1975.

It is expensive to build a new medical school as has been shown by recent experience at Hacettepe. It will also be difficult to get good faculty members to go to the smaller cities of Anatolia. The cost of building a medical school probably will be at least 10–15 million TL ($1,111,000–$1,666,000). The annual operating expenses will probably range over 20 million TL ($2,222,000). Alternative proposals for increasing the number of medical graduates must be carefully considered.

Summary Statement on Wastage of Medical Education Facilities

To get an indication of wasted medical school capacity, we calculated man-years spent in medical school from Table 3–52. Between 1947 and 1956, 24,898 student-years spent in medical school at Istanbul produced 2,531 graduates. In other words, if each student admitted to medical school had spent the minimum time of six years in school with no dropouts, the student-years spent would have been reduced to 15,186 or the graduates would have been increased to 4,150. Istanbul would have had a 64 percent increase in graduates. At Ankara 11,341 student-years could have been reduced to 7,368 student-years or an increase in number of graduates of 54 percent. For the two schools 36,239 man-years produced 3,759 graduates instead of a possible 6,040, a difference of 61 percent. Izmir and Hacettepe were too new to provide data.

The simplest way of increasing medical school output then would be to reduce dropouts and repeaters. It is estimated that the equivalent of two medical schools producing at least 115 graduates per year are now being lost in this way. The cost of two such schools will be at least 20–30 million TL in capital expenses and 40 million TL per year in operating expenses.

For a rapid increase of medical manpower, it is also possible to consider increasing the number of students per class in some of the existing medical schools. Newer innovations in teaching make such expansion feasible. Istanbul has for many years had such large classes that the institution should be split into two medical schools for optimum teaching. An appropriate balance must be maintained so that the classes do not become so large that the quality of education suffers. This hazard of overexpansion is particularly dangerous for the new educational experiments in producing community-oriented doctors which are being started at Hacettepe and Erzurum.

In summary, significant economies in medical education could be achieved by admitting only well-selected medical students who could profit from improved medical education and have a better prospect of graduating in the prescribed time.

Qualitative Description of Teaching Methods

Although quality of teaching is the most important determinant of medical education, it is also the most difficult to evaluate. No attempt will be made here to pass judgment on the quality of teaching in Turkey's medical schools. Some general statements will be made, however, about educational objectives in medicine and the teaching methods appropriate to achieving these objectives. With this background, a straightforward attempt will be made to describe the present patterns of teaching in Turkey.

Evaluation of teaching methods tends to be subjective and impressionistic because quantitative measures and valid standards have yet to be developed. In evaluating it is customary to concentrate on certain tangible qualities, such as knowledge and professional skill. More complex and ultimately more important are intangible qualities relating to the "art of medicine," such as ethical values and relationships with patients and colleagues.

Basic knowledge of facts and principles relating to health and disease has long been considered the major objective of medical education. At least this is clearly the focus of examination systems. The traditional didactic style of teaching developed empirically to provide maximum efficiency in communication during the centuries when professors served as the primary sources of knowledge. Progress in medical science has made traditional teaching methods obsolete. Medical knowledge is no longer a precious and limited flow to be carefully conserved and memorized from the educational pipeline of the professor's lectures and perhaps a single textbook, instead it has become a flood inundating the medical student. Rather than sipping from the fountain just enough to pass examinations and satisfy his intellectual needs, the student now has to swim desperately to stay afloat. Medical science has not only expanded beyond the capacity of any rational attempt to know everything but also is advancing so rapidly that what is learned in medical school becomes largely out-of-date ten years later.

A revolution in teaching methods has become necessary. The emphasis now is on student learning rather than on teaching. The role of the teacher in cognitive learning is primarily that of guiding the student in selecting what he should learn. In evaluating methods today, much more must be taken into account than knowledge acquired or examinations passed. More important is the question—how well have students learned to refer to the ever-changing sources of information and to think on their own?

A second tangible teaching objective is the student's acquisition of skills. These range from laboratory and clinical skills to those that determine effective personal relations. Evaluation techniques have long been available to test clinical skills but they usually involve personal observation to see how nearly the student can approximate the teacher's way of doing things. In learning skills the one essential requirement is that students must have the opportunity to practice under supervision. There should be built-in safeguards to keep them from learning wrong methods and they should have the chance to repeat correctly the complex processes required in medical practice until they become reflexive. The "practice" part of medicine must be provided for in the preparation of the doctor.

The third group of educational objectives is still largely intangible; attitudes, values, and interpersonal behavior are important considerations but we have little understanding of them. We do know that they are acquired primarily by imitation after personal contact with role models, among whom respected teachers have a dominant influence. The process of professionalization which eventually determines the distinguishing characteristics of doctors requires a set of group ethics and standard behavior patterns that are acceptable to colleagues and to society. These intangibles cannot be measured but they are too important to be left to chance. Students must have the opportunity to be closely associated with teachers who embody the desired attitudes and values.

In turning now to a description of teaching methods in Turkish medical schools, these three categories of objectives should be kept in mind. The transmission of knowledge, skills, and attitudes is discussed and an effort is made to frankly estimate limitations and areas of strength. It should be realized that there are notable exceptions to the generalizations which are made. When a broad pattern is described in terms which appear critical, it must be stressed that there are, of course, individual teachers and departments, or even whole schools, which do not fit into that pattern.

Most encouraging, is the recent trend of certain medical educators in Turkey to experiment with new and pioneering approaches which promise to radically change traditional medical education.

The pattern of medical education in Turkey is still strongly influenced by the German educational system of the past century which was at that time the best in the world. By today's standards, however, the teaching is much too didactic. The image of the great professor with a built-in aura of infallibility, as the source of all wisdom and knowledge, still pervades many clinical departments in Turkey. Such a system was excellent when medical knowledge was relatively static, in that information was transmitted directly, and with minimum dilution, from the professor to the students.

The limitations of the old system are increasingly obvious. Unless the professor himself is capable of initiating a whole flood of enquiry, innovative and research thinking will stagnate. Since the professor's status does not brook challenging, a spirit of free enquiry and questioning by subordinates is discouraged. Conformism has the usual rewards which come from gratifying the wishes and agreeing with the opinions of the chief of the clinic. Moreover, once the professor has reached his pedestal, the minimal pressure on him to maintain a fresh and inquisitive point of view leads to conservatism.

The most damaging aspect of overly didactic teaching is the effect it has on the medical student. It places a premium on theoretical learning—on ability to repeat the favorite dicta and opinions of the professor. Students leave medical school with a given quantum of information but without the continuing stimulus and the established intellectual habits needed to gain new knowledge.

The tendency toward large classes in some schools further emphasizes the essentially theoretical nature of the learning process. Most teaching is done by lecture and there is minimum opportunity for discussion. Even in day-to-day clinical teaching on ward rounds there is an all too common tendency for the teacher to lecture at the bedside, thus discouraging frank discussion. The patient serves only as a sounding board off whom lectures can be bounced. These bedside lectures may start with the professor expressing a somewhat dogmatic opinion about the diagnosis, oftentimes based on a single pet diagnostic maneuver. After the professor has spoken, there are few on the staff who will dare check the diagnosis with other appropriate tests.

In the teaching of skills, this pattern of didactic teaching is particularly defective. The student does not have chances to practice. This is partly due to serious shortages of laboratory equipment. Laboratory classes are often so handicapped by the lack of microscopes and other equipment that long cues of students line up behind demonstrations for a few seconds of peering at a parasitic ovum, a bacterial smear, or a simple chemical test. In clinical wards opportunities to practice under supervision are almost nonexistent because of the competition for access to patients among residents who are being trained as specialists.

Among the important intangible factors affecting attitude and value development, the greatest obstacle is the large gap between teachers and students. The high position of the professor removes him from the easy contact with students that is required for optimum professionalization. To the student the professor remains a remote figure whose values are represented mainly by material indices of success, such as a prestigious automobile.

The somewhat extreme picture thus far presented is all too typical of much of the medical education in Turkey. On the other hand, there are some notable changes underway. In some institutions, and in some departments, encouraging strides are being made in pioneering new approaches to medical education. Not only is good use being made of new information about educational methodology, but also new experiments are being conducted which may well lead to innovations in medical education that will be important demonstrations for the whole world. This new and experimental approach thus far has been most evident in the new schools which tend to draw the young and imaginative medical educators.

Specific Changes in Medical Education Required to Meet Modern Demands

a. The teaching of basic sciences must be revised. Rather than teaching minutiae of anatomy and enzymology which are promptly forgotten, the emphasis should be on what is practical and usable in medical practice. Those doctors who go into research can learn the details of their specialty basic sciences as part of their research training. Most imperative is a thorough indoctrination in the scientific point of view. The student must understand basic principles well enough to develop the habits of problem-solving so much needed in understanding shifting patterns of disease.

b. Most important are the subtle changes needed to deliberately channel the influences which medical educators can have on the attitudes and motivations of medical students. Values instilled in medical students as part of the process of professionalization are usually acquired from highly respected teachers. To be an adequate role model to his students, the professor must demonstrate in his own day-to-day activities the sort of professional example which society expects of doctors.

  c. The central focus of the Turkish doctors' attention in the future should be his responsibility to the community. The premedical and preclinical portions of medical education should, therefore, include basic sciences which are devoted especially to understanding groups rather than concentrating only on individuals. Particular stress should be placed on the social sciences, statistics, and, most of all, epidemiology. Students must also be given a chance to appreciate fundamental concepts underlying human relations, subjects such as genetics and the ways in which growth and development influence behavior.

  d. Clinical preparation must focus on the whole patient. It should be practical with primary stress on clinical skills which will make efficient, effective, and economic diagnosis and treatment the routine. Because the family and community approach is so important in the new planning for comprehensive care, a major part of clinical preparation should be in regionalized practice areas where total care can be demonstrated. Sound experience with the common diseases of the area is absolutely essential, especially where infectious and nutritional health problems are important.

  e. Since rural practice is the greatest unmet need in Turkey, doctors should be specifically prepared for such responsibility. This requires an exposure to rural units where comprehensive clinical work is practiced by specialists in rural medicine. The teachers must personally typify the best qualities of a practicing community doctor. Rural teaching should emphasize the team approach and show how a doctor can expand his capacity for service by working through auxiliaries.

  f. Permeating the new approach to medical education should be a much greater emphasis on preventive services. The health needs of Turkey will never be met by curative activities alone. All doctors must co-operate in applying preventive principles in work with the individual, the family, and the community.

REFERENCES

1. *Cumburiyet Dauri Saglik Bareketler: (Health Activities in Republican Era) 1923–63* (1964).
2. Government of Turkey, *Official Annual Budget*, 1954–64, incl.

4

SUPPLY OF NURSES

By Alice M. Forman

Nursing in Turkey appears to be entering a long overdue period of development. No part of direct health services has been more neglected. No other category of health personnel is in as short supply as trained nurses. There are at least five doctors for every registered nurse. Behind the present shortage is a complex historical tradition.

In Turkey, nursing has not been regarded generally as a profession but as menial employment for women of low social status and prestige. In order to improve the image of nursing and also to meet the pressing need for trained supervisors and administrators, registered nurses have tended to concentrate on high-level functions such as supervision and administration rather than on direct patient care. Most patients never see a registered nurse. Even in the better hospitals direct patient care is provided mainly by *hastabakici* or "patient helpers" who have had little or no education and only on-the-job training. The costly scientific education of doctors is often wasted because they must supervise patient care provided by auxiliaries, undertake nursing care of the critically ill and deal with details of nursing administration.

Responsible government officials have repeatedly expressed their concern about the shortage of professional nurses in hospitals and public health services, especially since the end of World War II. Many efforts by government, voluntary groups, and international agencies to improve the situation have made people more aware of the problem and generated pressure to seek for solutions. The number of graduates from Turkish nursing schools has increased, but public demands for improved nursing services have increased more rapidly. Proposed expansion and improvement of hospital and public health services are likely to remain mere paper plans unless sufficient nurses are prepared to share in their implementation.

Our study of nursing in Turkey started during the summer of 1963 with an informal preliminary survey. It included interviews with nurses and doctors in key positions, a review of official documents and previous studies, and direct observations. Subjective impressions and partial data suggested clues to the nature of the nurse supply problem in Turkey. Not only was recruitment of candidates inadequate but there were reports of a general tendency for graduates to rapidly leave professional activities. One doctor in a teaching and research center said, "After nurses are trained, they vanish." Directors of hospital nursing services gave the more realistic explanation that most married nurses were unable to continue working because twelve hours of duty was expected for six to seven days a week and no special allowances were paid to those living outside of hospitals. Directors of nursing schools also stated that a large number of nurses were leaving Turkey to work abroad because of better salaries and accommodations and, especially, because of more favorable attitudes of doctors and the public toward nurses. In contrast, Ministry of Health data indicated that 86 percent of the nurses registered with the Ministry of Health were actively employed in Turkey. It was said that in many institutions the budgeted positions for registered nurses were used for nurses' aides or laboratory technicians, less because of the lack of registered nurses than because trained nurses' aides were cheaper and because doctors preferred to employ technicians for laboratory work. Some positions budgeted for directors of nursing were used for doctors doing medical research or for university instructors in the humanities. Behind these statements loomed the obvious fact that many doctors did not really respect nurses or know how to make the best use of their services.

As in other countries where intensive efforts are being made to meet increasing demands for nursing services, so also in Turkey there is a confusing patchwork of different categories of health personnel and training programs. The varied experiences in Turkey are not so much experiments as trial and error efforts to meet the changing qualitative and quantitative demands for nursing services in a developing country. Popular demand increases both because of greater sophistication and population growth. This rising tide of demand has led to ambitious programs such as the nationalization of health services. The need for realistic and imaginative planning and priority setting is nowhere more evident than in defining the role of nurses in the health manpower balance.

This chapter reviews briefly the historical development of nursing in Turkey, categories of nursing personnel, educational programs for nursing, characteristics of the present supply of registered nurses, trends in the supply, and considerations for planning future supply.

HISTORICAL BACKGROUND

Nursing in Turkey has a fairly recent history, especially as compared with medicine. The first registered nurses graduated from the Red Crescent School of Nursing in Istanbul in 1927, less than forty years ago and more than sixty-five years after Florence Nightingale established the first organized school of nursing in London. This cultural lag was related to the general attitude toward careers for women in traditional Muslim society; there was little respect for women who worked and near-condemnation of women who ministered to strangers—especially men—even though they were sick.

The status of women changed conspicuously when Turkey became a republic in 1923. Major reforms included unveiling, compulsory secular education, and co-education. The first Turkish nursing school graduated nurses in the same year that the first group of women doctors graduated from the University of Istanbul.

Nursing began to be recognized as a profession even more recently. The difficult adjustments have included timing problems such as the starting of university-level nursing programs before enough positions were available for the new graduates. Similarly, auxiliary nurse-training programs were established without defining clear differences in responsibilities and privileges between trained nurse auxiliaries and registered nurses. Other problems concerned professional control of nursing. In 1954, a law was passed to regulate nursing education and practice. Although this law stipulates that only graduates of schools approved by the Ministry are to be employed as graduate nurses, strict adherence to this stipulation has proved difficult, due to the shortage of registered nurses.

With WHO assistance, an effort was made to raise the status of nursing nationally through the establishment of a Bureau of Nursing in the Ministry of Health and the formation of an Advisory Council on Nursing. As nursing education programs increased numerically and in importance, there continued to be an obvious failure to use experienced Turkish nurse educators in official planning for the development of nursing services. Improvement in the supply and utilization of nurses has been hampered by diffusion of responsibility for nursing. Various directorates in the Ministry of Health deal more or less independently with training, licensure, assignments, and working conditions. With the exception of the General Directorate of Professional Education and Training, none of the health directorates at national or provincial levels has even now appointed professional nurses to its administrative staff.

The Turkish Nurses' Assocation has tried more or less unsuccessfully to modify national policy. The Nurses' Association's recommendations of 1963, based on the experience of professional nursing groups in Turkey and in other countries, have received little attention from the Ministry of Health.

In spite of these problems, it is remarkable that in only four decades nursing has approached professional standing in Turkey. This is considerably faster than the rate at which nursing was accepted professionally in Europe. Turkish nurses now obtain university diplomas and hold responsible positions in hospitals and as directors in schools of nursing. They are beginning to serve in official and advisory capacities in the government.

However, this acceptance has extended to only a relatively small group of nurses thus far. Most women identified as "nurses" are essentially uneducated or untrained for their specific tasks. The long-standing stigma attached to nursing continues to influence recruitment unfavorably. This recruitment problem may get worse as Turkey's progressive modernization makes other occupations available to women.

METHODOLOGY OF THE STUDY

Surveys of nursing services in Turkey have in the past tended to be partial and focused on special subjects such as role perceptions of nurses[1] or the establishment of university-level schools of nursing.[2] Our study in 1964–65 was an attempt to get a complete definition of the distribution, characteristics, and career patterns of nurses who were the counterparts of professional nurses in other countries.[3]

The sample for the study was selected from all nurses trained in Turkey from 1927 to 1963 in schools preparing registered nurses, nurse-midwives, or midwives. The schools included were all those recognized by the Ministry of Health as preparing these three types of personnel, since graduates of these schools are usually appointed as nurses. A random sample of 817 was selected from the 2,692 graduates of the fourteen schools meeting the criteria of the study.

Tracing these individuals was difficult and time-consuming because of frequent changes in surnames, primarily due to marriage. The staff of the nursing schools proved to be the best sources of information. Also effective were the contacts nurses maintained through social communications with classmates. A series of teas was organized to bring such social groups together. Within a period of eight months about 85 percent were traced as to whether they were living or dead, and their place of residence. Detailed information was obtained from these nurses by means of personal interviews and mailed questionnaires.

In addition, background information on staffing patterns in hospitals, student enrollments, and teaching staff in nursing schools was obtained through questionnaires mailed directly to the institutions. Descriptions of nursing curricula, nursing laws and regulations were provided by the Ministry of Health.

CATEGORIES OF NURSING PERSONNEL

Unplanned proliferation of many types of training programs has resulted in numerous categories of health workers who perform nursing functions. Each category is listed in the public health laws, with overlapping regulations about training and functions, but the differences between them and their interrelationships are not clear. Important among these categories is the *saglik memuru* (see Chapter 5), a general purpose male worker trained to carry out some of the functions of public health nurses in mass disease control campaigns and often used as a clinical auxiliary. Another major category is the trained assistant nurse or nurse's aide who often substitutes directly for a registered nurse. The numerical distributions in these categories are determined mainly by the size of the pool of educated persons available for training. More men than women with eight years of schooling were available for training in public health work and large numbers of *saglik memurus* resulted. Among women the educational pool was shallow after primary school with the result that the practical nurse aide expanded rapidly because of the availability of this educational level.

The major categories of personnel involved in nursing fall into two main groups. One includes the personnel trained at lycee or university levels (Table 4–1), whereas the other consists of health workers trained at the middle-school level or below (Table 4–2).

Registered Nurses (Hemsire)

Registered nurses include two levels of training both qualified to be registered by the Ministry of Health, the lycee-level and the university-level nurses. Although lycee-level nurses make up the large majority of registered nurses, they are actually more nearly equivalent in education to the assistant nurse or licensed practical nurse in Western countries. Little distinction is made in official listing of the functions and responsibilities of lycee- and university-level nurses. On the other hand, their salaries begin at different levels according to the Turkish government's scale based on stages of education completed. Also, opportunities for advanced professional education are more readily available to the university-level graduate nurse. A lycee-level graduate nurse may qualify for admission to a master's level program of study only after she has passed the regular lycee examination and then obtained a university diploma.

Professional Midwives (Ebe)

Most of the urban midwives take only a two-year program of training. However, it is anticipated that the numbers of nurse-midwives who receive four years' training, including general nursing, will progressively increase. This trend is appropriate because nurse-midwives are often substituted for nurses in supervision of general nursing services as well as maternity care.

Saglik Memuru

As described in Chapter 5, *saglik memurus* are men who usually have not been included in nursing studies because their training has not included bedside nursing and their experience has been mainly in community health activities. The relationship with nursing will be intensified because the first three years of their training in health colleges is being co-ordinated with that of nurses. The three-year post-basic program at Gevher Nesibe Institute is open to *saglik memurus* as well as nurses. Graduates from both backgrounds are assigned to be teachers and administrators in health colleges and health schools. As *saglik memurus* increasingly fill key positions in nursing education and administration, the development of nursing may be handicapped because of their lack of preparation and interest in bedside nursing. Furthermore, if *saglik memurus* are to continue to be influential in nursing services the scope of their work, like that of nurses, must be controlled by public laws.

Nursing Instructor

Two types of training qualify nurses as instructors: completion of the three-year post-basic program at Gevher Nesibe Higher Institute, and obtaining a bachelor's or master's degree in nursing. In 1964, a new public health law raised the status and emoluments for graduates of Gevher Nesibe to that of other professional teachers in health colleges and health schools.

Assistant Nurses or Nurses' Aides (Hemsire Yardimcisi)

No examination or licensure is required for these women. They have only five years' general education and two years' hospital training in nursing but serve as equivalent to registered nurses in many hospitals and rural health centers. Instead of working under the supervision of registered nurses they are often solely responsible for nursing services. Since nurses' aides are more in evidence in wards and clinics than are registered nurses, their behavior in daily personal contacts with patients and doctors has an important and sometimes detrimental effect on the image of nurses in general. Few nurses' aides seek to become better qualified in nursing because the only route for them to advance is by taking the recognized training programs for registered nurses, which requires the investment of an additional seven years in education.

Village Midwives (Koyebesi)

After five years of primary education these women receive three years' training in maternity hospitals. The present curriculum in health schools is also designed to teach them simple nursing as well as maternal and child health services. In the new nationalized health services they are scheduled to have an important role in providing direct services to village families. In rural stiuations the acceptance of these midwives is hampered because they are often young, under twenty years of age, and have little access to professional supervision and guidance. It is almost anachronistic that

TABLE 4–1. MAIN CATEGORIES OF NURSING AND MIDWIFERY PERSONNEL TRAINED IN LYCEE-LEVEL AND UNIVERSITY-LEVEL PROGRAMS IN TURKEY, 1964

Designation	Place of employment	Functions	General education required (years)	Professional or technical training programs	Length of training (years)
Registered nurse (*Hemsire*)	Hospitals. Urban training centers for nurses and assistant nurses. Health schools for rural midwives.	Mainly administration, teaching, and supervision of auxiliary nursing personnel and rural midwives.	8	Health college programs sponsored by Ministry of Health. Nursing school programs sponsored by voluntary agencies.	4
			11	University-level programs at Ankara University, Ege University, Florence Nightingale College of Nursing.	4

Midwife (*Ebe*)	Maternity hospitals and MCH centers in cities. Schools for rural midwives.	Care of mothers before, during, and after labor. Teaching and supervision of rural midwives. Private practice.	8	Program conducted by Istanbul University Faculty of Medicine.	2
Nurse midwife	(Same as for midwife)	(Same as for midwife)	8	Two health colleges sponsored by Ministry of Health offer programs combining midwifery with general nursing.	4
Saglik memuru (Sanitarian health officer, male nurse, health technician)	Rural health centers. T.B., V.D., and malaria control programs.	Simple diagnostic laboratory procedures. Treatment of patients. Health education. Supervision of auxiliaries. Clerical and statistical work.	8	Training in health colleges along with female professional nursing personnel. Choices in major areas of study include male nursing for psychiatric institutions, x-ray technology, laboratory technology, environmental sanitation.	4

TABLE 4–2. MAIN CATEGORIES OF NURSING AND MIDWIFERY PERSONNEL TRAINED AT MIDDLE-SCHOOL LEVEL OR BELOW IN TURKEY, 1964

Designation	Place of employment	Functions	General education required (years)	Professional or technical training programs	Length of training (years)
Practical nurse, trained assistant nurse, trained nurse's aide. (*Hemsire yardimcisi*)	Hospitals and rural health centers.	Bedside nursing. Administration of ward or clinic nursing services and supervision of hospital aides where there are no registered nurses.	5	Apprenticeship training in 51 general hospitals in cities. Minimum age requirement is 18 years.	2

Title	Place of employment	Functions		Training	
Village midwife (*Köyebesi*)	MCH or PH centers in rural areas, primarily; also, in urban MCH centers. Occasionally in rural and urban homes.	Maternity service and child health care. Supervised by public health nurse and midwife. Assists in family health services, in clinics and home visiting. Occasionally private practice. *Note:* Scope of functions depends on training and supervision.	5	Combined nursing and midwifery programs in health schools connected with maternity hospitals. Refresher courses of 2–4 weeks sponsored by Ministry of Health, WHO, and UNICEF. Each midwife expected to attend one refresher course annually.	3
Hospital aide or nurse's aide or orderly (*Hastabakici*)	Hospitals	Housekeeping and simple patient care under supervision of trained nurse or nurse's aide. Does technical nursing under supervision of doctors in places employing no trained nurses.	None	No formal training.	

only after they have completed six years of service in villages are they eligible to work in urban centers where professional assistance is more readily available.

Hospital Aides (Hastabakici)

Both men and women are employed as hospital aides (literally translated "patient helper") without regard to educational background. They learn from experience on the job. Generally they have more contact with patients than trained personnel and provide much of the direct patient care without direct supervision from nurses. The lack of regulations concerning their responsibilities and training means that their activities range from simple housekeeping tasks and patient care to administration of anesthetics in hospital operating rooms.

One Turkish health official aptly described the unstructured personnel pattern for nursing and midwifery services when he said that anyone wearing a white uniform and caring for a patient is apt to be addressed—and viewed—as *hemsire* by physicians, other hospital staff, and the public. This dilution of the title of nurse suggests that extreme measures may be necessary, including perhaps the introduction of a completely new set of respectable professional titles which can be clearly distinguished.

RELATIVE SIZES OF CATEGORIES

Some idea of the numerical importance of the various types of nursing personnel is obtained from the over-all data on staffing patterns of hospitals sponsored by different agencies included in our 1964 institutional survey.

In 241 general and special hospitals with 34,345 beds, sponsored by the Ministry of Health only, the over-all ratio of all trained nursing and midwifery personnel (including *saglik memurus*, nurses, assistant nurses, midwives, and rural midwives) to physicians was 1.02 per physician. The total of 1,872 trained personnel providing nursing services in these hospitals was distributed as follows:

Saglik memurus	5.0 percent
Nurses	34.2 percent
Assistant nurses	55.3 percent
Midwives	2.6 percent
Rural midwives	2.9 percent

The number of untrained *hastabakicis* was not reported, but in those institutions visited by members of our team they were always reported to be "many" and they were certainly most in evidence on hospital wards.

Some concrete examples of the extensive use of untrained *hastabakicis* were obtained from reports of thirty-one general hospitals with over 3,000 beds sponsored by other ministries, agencies, medical schools, and state economic enterprises. Other than physicians, dentists, and pharmacists, the 1,235 hospital personnel were distributed as follows: nurses 7.7 percent, nurse aides 6.3 percent, other personnel 86.0 percent. The "other personnel" consisted mostly of *hastabakicis* who, with few exceptions, provided the patient care services.

PROFESSIONAL EDUCATION OF REGISTERED NURSES

In the forty years since the first Turkish school of nursing opened, basic training for nursing has changed from two-year hospital-based programs for girls with primary school education (five years) to four-year programs in independent educational institutions for girls who have completed middle school (three years) or lycee (three years). Post-basic nursing programs are at the level of technical and teacher training institutes outside the universities. The rapid multiplication of schools is indicated by the fact that fourteen basic nursing programs at both lycee level (post middle school) and university level (post lycee) were opened between 1961 and 1963.

By 1964, twenty-six institutions in Turkey were providing basic nurses' training. Of the lycee-level schools, twenty were health colleges sponsored by the Ministry of Health and three were conducted by private or semi-private agencies (Table 4–3). There were three higher schools of nursing at the university level. In addition, one institution offered post-basic education for nurses, as well as *saglik memurus* and midwives. By 1965, two more lycee-level schools had opened. These were not included in Table 4–3 because enrollment figures were not available.

More than half of the active nurses in 1964 were graduates of schools sponsored by the Ministry of Health. The educational qualifications of the active nurses in the 1964 survey suggests that their preparation was primarily vocational rather than professional. Only 9 percent of these respondents had completed secondary school. Less than 16 percent had any form of postbasic education

TABLE 4–3. SELECTED CHARACTERISTICS OF LYCEE-LEVEL PROGRAMS FOR NURSES IN TURKEY IN 1964–5, ACCORDING TO SPONSORING AGENCIES

Number of institutions	Duration of program (years)	Current enrollment			Total graduates to end of 1963			Resident status of students
		Female	Male	Total	Female	Male	Total	
Voluntary agencies 3	3–4	317	—	317	1,206	—	1,206	Boarding only
Ministry of Health 20	4	1,142	1,792	2,934	1,335	2,154	3,489	Day and boarding
Totals 23	—	1,459	1,792	3,251	2,541	2,154	4,695	—

in either nursing or other fields. Only 9.2 percent had had experience or education abroad. Although the majority of active nurses in Turkey have administrative, supervisory, or teaching responsibilities, it is evident that relatively few have been adequately prepared for these duties.

Health Colleges

Health colleges are independent educational institutions which have four-year basic nursing programs for men and women who have completed at least a middle school education of eight years. The average age on admission is sixteen years. In mid-1964, fourteen of the colleges were either co-educational or all male, while only six, including midwifery colleges, admitted only women. Nurses receive practical training in general nursing in affiliated hospitals and rural health centers and nurse-midwives receive maternity training in hospitals. The broad curriculum provides both a basic science foundation and practical experience in nursing. Graduates have the same government pay scales as lycee graduates although they are not qualified for admission to a university. All nurses are given some instruction in methods of teaching and administration because after graduation many are employed as teachers in the rapidly expanding schools for rural midwives.

Although the rationale for the recently inaugurated health college curriculum recommended by the Turkish Ministry of Health appears sound, initial experiences of several health colleges have revealed problems which will have to be overcome. A crucial difficulty is that student nurses and staff are having to cope simultaneously with two almost full-time curricula—traditional nurse training and current lycee education. Effective amalgamation of the two is difficult for at least three important reasons. First, health college students are largely those who have not been able to cope satisfactorily with lycee courses. Second, the teaching staff of health colleges usually includes large numbers of part-time people who have multiple teaching responsibilities in a variety of institutions including some unrelated to nursing. This leads to fragmentation and irrelevancy in what is taught student nurses. Third, health colleges generally have no control over the quality of practical experiences provided for students in hospitals. Inadequate practical preparation for nursing results because hospitals are staffed mainly by auxiliary personnel with the limited professional staff being preoccupied with service responsibilities.

Costs of nursing education are borne by the Ministry of Health, which provides tuition, room, board, uniforms and pocket money for resident students. Nonresidents must pay their own living expenses. In return for their education, graduates who have been residents must serve in Ministry of Health institutions for at least five years following graduation.

Lycee-Level Schools of Nursing

In 1964, three schools of nursing under non- or quasi-government auspices were recognized by the Ministry of Health. Female students with eight years of general education undertake a four-year program similar to that in the health colleges. One school has a three-year curriculum for nurses in tuberculosis control programs. Many students graduate before they are twenty years old and their compulsory service terms vary from none up to four years.

University-Level Schools of Nursing

Each of the three main metropolitan cities of Turkey has a government-sponsored university-level school of nursing, admitting lycee graduates and offering a four-year basic nursing program. They differ in several respects—age, size, curriculum, recognition for graduates, and compulsory service required.

Ege University School of Nursing and Medical Technicians in Izmir was opened in 1955 but had graduated only nine nurses by the end of 1964 when enrollment was sixteen female and seventeen male students. The Florence Nightingale College of Nursing in Istanbul and the Ankara University School of Nursing, which opened in 1961, had enrollments of forty-three and seventy-five respectively by 1964. By 1965 the total number of graduates was twenty-three. Hacettepe School of Nursing started university-level teaching in 1964. Policy variations range from the Florence Nightingale College's arrangement for awarding a diploma that is not recognized as a university degree but with graduates committed to serve the Ministry of Health for eight years, to the Ankara University School of Nursing being able to grant a university diploma with only three years' compulsory service after graduation.

All schools include practical work but the kinds and amounts vary. Florence Nightingale College is attempting to develop good public health nursing experience in a recently organized health center; however, it is handicapped in providing consistently good hospital nursing experience because of inadequate hospital affiliations. Ankara University School of Nursing has arranged for limited public health experience in a social pediatrics clinic. Considerable supervised clinical nursing experience is provided at Hacettepe. Ege University, with a combined study program for nurses and medical technicians, has given comparatively little attention to effective nursing experience in hospitals and public health activities.

Post-Basic Education Programs

In Ankara the Gevher Nesibe Higher Institute of Health Education opened in 1961 under the sponsorship of the Ministry of Health. The three-year programs prepare nurses, midwives, and *saglik memurus* who have completed lycee-level training for teaching in health colleges and health schools, and for "middle-level administration" in public health and hospital services. By 1965 Gevher Nesibe graduates totaled 45 and enrollment had reached 103 with a majority (60 percent) being *saglik memurus*.

It is already evident that future complications will occur unless interrelationships between the universities and the Ministry of Health can be improved. Graduates of the Florence Nightingale College of Nursing and Gevher Nesibe Higher Institute will probably not qualify for master's or doctor's degrees in universities in Turkey and other countries. Conversely the Ministry of Health has had only limited influence in establishing adequate standards for practical experience in clinical and public health work.

SUPPLY OF NURSES

It is estimated that of the 2,963 women graduated from professional nursing schools during the period 1927–64, about 1,852 (62.5 percent) were actively engaged in nursing in Turkey in 1964. The inactive group is estimated to be 797 (26.9 percent) living in Turkey, with an additional 92 (3.1 percent) deceased and 222 (7.5 percent) living abroad.

DISTRIBUTION OF ACTIVE NURSES

In the country as a whole in 1964 there were approximately 16,538 persons per registered nurse, or about six nurses per 100,000 population. Regional ratios varied from one nurse for 4,817 population in the European region of Turkey to one nurse for 87,800 people in southeastern Anatolia. Table 4–4 shows the gross imbalances in the distribution of registered nurses as compared with population in the eight geographic regions of Turkey. Turkey in Europe contains only about 10 percent of the population, but employs approximately 34 percent of the active nurses.

TABLE 4–4. ACTIVE NURSE SUPPLY COMPARED WITH POPULATION, HOSPITAL BEDS, AND DOCTORS IN EIGHT REGIONS OF TURKEY IN 1964

	Percent distribution			Ratios	
Regions	Active nurses (N=1,852)	Population (N= 30,628,892)	Hospital beds (N=74,506)	Beds per nurse	Doctors per nurse
Turkey in Europe	33.7	9.8	28.8	34.4	6.3
Black Sea coast	5.4	16.0	7.4	55.4	5.5
Marmara and Aegean Sea coasts	15.2	16.1	17.1	45.2	5.2
Mediterranean Sea coast	3.0	7.6	4.1	54.4	8.4
Western Anatolia	4.6	8.5	7.9	69.1	4.6
Central Anatolia	30.5	24.8	22.3	29.4	4.5
Southeast Anatolia	0.8	4.3	2.0	100.3	10.6
Eastern Anatolia	6.8	12.9	10.4	61.5	3.6
All regions	100.0	100.0	100.0	40.2	5.4

The concentration of nurses in the three metropolitan areas is more clearly presented in Table 4–5, where they are shown to be even more urban than physicians. As long as most professional nurses continue to be used for educational and administrative functions, a distribution of this sort is to be expected. As schools are started in other areas, a more even distribution should result.

TABLE 4–5. PERCENT DISTRIBUTION OF ACTIVE NURSES, PHYSICIANS, AND POPULATION BY TYPE OF COMMUNITY

Type of community	Active nurses	Practicing physicians	Population
Villages and towns	9.6	13.4	68.1
Cities	26.5	25.2	26.8
Metropolitan areas	63.9	61.4	5.1
Total	100.0	100.0	100.0

Perhaps the most dramatic single statistic illustrating the shortage of nurses is the simple discovery that there are at least five doctors for every registered nurse. This is the reverse of the ratio usually aimed for in most countries. East Anatolia, where the new national-ization of health services program had been in operation for one year, had the lowest ratio (about four doctors/nurse) (Table 4–4). Southeast Anatolia, with similar conditions but no nationalization program, had the highest doctor-nurse ratio, about eleven doctors per nurse.

Although there is a general association, the shortage of registered nurses is not directly correlated with the distribution of hospital beds (Table 4–4). This is not suprising since nurses perform little direct patient care. Ratios of beds to nurses are most favorable in metropolitan areas. Ankara (Central Anatolia) has the lowest ratio, since it has multiple large hospitals, with Hacettepe having a particularly large staff of registered nurses. Southeast Anatolia has only one nurse for one-hundred beds.

Most of the active nurses in Turkey are employed in the public sector (about 89 percent). The Ministry of Health, including provincial governments and municipal health departments, em-ploys the largest proportion (approximately 51 percent). Among the nongovernmental agencies, philanthropic institutions have the largest proportion (about 9 percent) of the employed registered nurses with only a handful of nurses being self-employed or in-dependent.

On the other hand, although the Ministry of Health supports a majority of the hospital beds and employs the largest proportion of nurses, its over-all bed-nurse ratio is less favorable than the ratios in hospitals supported by other government agencies (Table 4–6). The most favorable bed-nurse ratio was in hospitals sponsored by philanthropic agencies.

A large majority of active nurses are employed in service institu-tions such as hospitals, sanatoria, and health centers (87 percent). Eight percent are on the teaching staff of nursing and midwifery schools and another 5 percent are in other types of institutions, including laboratories and the Bureau of Nursing in the Ministry of Health. The 1964 nursing study showed that most registered nurses were working in administrative and supervisory positions in nursing services (58 percent) and only about one-third worked as staff nurses. The number of nurses actually engaged in patient care was undoubtedly considerably lower judging from responses to questions in the sample survey about their work. Even the lowest

TABLE 4–6. NUMBER OF HOSPITAL BEDS AND NURSES AND NURSE/BED RATIOS IN HOSPITALS SPONSORED BY GOVERNMENT AGENCIES, BASED ON 1964 SAMPLE OF NURSES

Type of administration	Total number of hospital beds	Estimated number of nurses	Number of beds per nurse
Ministry of Health	40,785	937	43.5
Other ministries, state economic enterprises, medical schools	18,709	563	33.2
Government workers insurance	4,176	146	28.6

of these figures exaggerates the number of nurses available for hospitals because the calculations do not exclude nurses employed in the 331 dispensaries and health centers without beds or in the Health Ministry's 47 training institutions for nursing and midwifery personnel.

ACTIVITY PATTERNS OF NURSES

In order to have some idea of the work patterns of nurses during the years following graduation, a curve was constructed by applying over time the 1964 activity rates obtained in the cross-sectional study of a sample of nurses. These activity rates, by each graduation year, included in the numerator nurses who reported themselves as active at the time of the study and in the denominator all in the sample who were graduated the same year. It was assumed that those who did not respond to the survey questionnaire were inactive. The rates were smoothed to form a distinct bimodal curve (Figure 4–1). Even with obvious understatement of activity rates obtained by this method, it is impressive that over-all activity rates are as high as 66 percent in comparison with other countries such as the United States where the over-all activity rate for professional nurses is estimated to be about 50 percent.[4]

The activity curve indicates that graduates leave nursing at the rate of 5–6 percent per year for the first ten years following graduation. The low point of about 41 percent remaining active in nursing is reached about twelve years after graduation. Nurses then tend to return to nursing in increasing numbers for the next eight or nine years up to a level of 66 percent active, after which the percent who are active again diminishes.

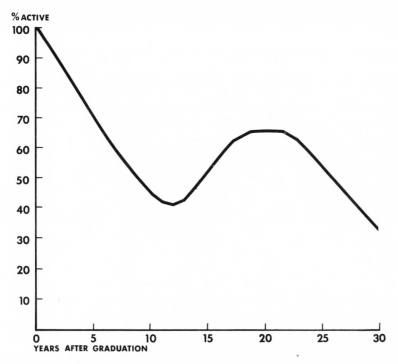

FIGURE 4–1. ESTIMATED PERCENT OF REGISTERED NURSES ACTIVELY EMPLOYED IN
NURSING BY THE INTERVAL AFTER GRADUATION.

Factors Influencing Active Nurse Supply

The trend for a certain proportion of nurses to return to nursing
after periods of inactivity is illustrated also by the different age
distributions when the 656 respondents were classified in three
career groups: (a) continuously active in nursing in Turkey; (b)
presently active but not continuously active in the past (intermittently active); and (c) presently inactive (Figure 4–2). This last
group includes those who never worked, those who may have
worked intermittently in the past, and those living abroad. The
majority of those in the continuously active group are young and
recent graduates, while the majority of intermittently active and
inactive are over thirty years of age. This age distribution strongly
suggests that whether or not a nurse is actively working in nursing
is closely related to her age.

Marriage and child-rearing are probably the main reasons for
temporary or permanent withdrawal from nursing. Of 656 respondents in the 1964 study approximately 50 percent were married.

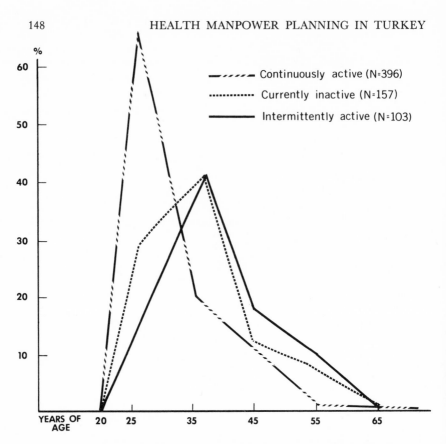

FIGURE 4–2. AGE DISTRIBUTION OF GROUPS OF REGISTERED NURSES BY PATTERN
OF NURSING EMPLOYMENT REPORTED IN THEIR WORK HISTORIES.

Table 4–7 shows clearly that married women tended to be those
who were no longer active in nursing.

TABLE 4–7. MARITAL STATUS OF NURSES CONTINUOUSLY ACTIVE, INTERMITTENTLY
ACTIVE, AND INACTIVE, BY PERCENT, IN 1964

	Total (N=656)	Continuously active (N=396)	Intermittently active (N=103)	Inactive in Turkey (N=157)
Single	49.3	68.1	27.2	16.6
Married	44.6	28.4	56.3	77.7
Widowed	2.1	1.5	2.9	3.2
Divorced	4.0	2.0	13.6	2.5
Total	100.0	100.0	100.0	100.0

Married nurses without children are also likely to remain in nursing but when married nurses have children the age patterns of their families appear to be more important than the numbers of children in determining activity (Table 4–8). The average number of children for 198 active married respondents was 1.1 whereas the 130 inactive married respondents had an average of 1.4 children. Only 1.5 percent of all married respondents had more than 3 children. Responses of 326 married nurses in the special study indicated that when their children were of school age, they were most likely to be inactive (Table 4–8). But when they had one or more preschool children or infants, over 60 percent continued working.

TABLE 4–8. PERCENT DISTRIBUTION BY ACTIVITY STATUS OF 326 MARRIED NURSES*
ACCORDING TO THE AGE PATTERNS OF THEIR CHILDREN IN 1964

Ages of children	Continuously active	Intermittently active	Inactive in Turkey	Total number
No children	49.3	28.0	22.7	75 (100%)
One or more under 7 years	44.4	15.9	39.7	126 (100%)
All school age and over	26.6	21.1	52.3	109 (100%)
All children 18 years of age or older	12.5	50.0	37.5	16 (100%)

*Includes widowed and divorced. Excludes 6 married nurses who did not give information about children.

The unexpected discovery that Turkish nurses tend to work when they have small children suggests that other factors intrinsic to marriage determine whether or not married nurses work. Economic need and husband's social status appear to be important as revealed by developing profiles of the three career groups of nurses.

Profiles of Nurse Career Groups

The *continuously active* group was young (about 67 percent under twenty-nine), usually single (68 percent), and childless (only 22 percent had children). Of the nurses with families, most of the children were very young. Nearly half of these women had grown up in villages and small towns. Over 50 percent of their husbands were in technical fields and over a third were professional workers with university preparation.

Intermittently active nurses were older (74 percent were thirty or more), usually married (75 percent were or had been married), and over half (52 percent) had children. Husbands of this group were most often white collar or professional workers (40 percent were employed in professions). Few husbands were unemployed. Only 29 percent of these nurses were from villages and towns.

Inactive nurses were usually still in a child-rearing age group; only a third were over forty. Eighty-three percent were married, and 86 percent of those married had children. Only 29 percent were from villages and towns. The socioeconomic status of this group, as evidenced by husbands' employment, was significantly higher than in the other groups. Sixty-five percent of the husbands had higher education, and 69 percent held responsible administrative positions or were in professions. The proportion of nurses in the inactive group married to physicians (32 percent) was three times that of the intermittently active group (11 percent) and four times that of the continuously active group (8 percent). This suggests that nurse-physician marriages contribute to the wife's leaving active nursing.

The rapid expansion of nursing schools means that there is now a preponderance of young nurses. Since 50 percent of nurses were under thirty years of age and 82 percent were less than forty years, activity levels may drop somewhat unless nursing education continues to expand. The large number of young and inexperienced nurses may lower the quality of nursing services because of a lack of mature nurses for supervision and administration in hospitals.

The over-all percentage of nurses who spent their childhood in rural areas was thirty-eight. During the past ten years the trend has been toward an increasing proportion of recruits from these areas. This coincides with increased opportunities for girls to be educated in rural areas and with expansion of health services in these areas. The fact that a much larger percentage of *always active* nurses were from rural areas is an encouraging sign.

UTILIZATION OF NURSES

The most readily available and rapidly applicable means of increasing nursing services is to improve utilization of the present nursing force. Increasing the output of nursing schools alone requires considerable time and financial investment. There have been no definitive nurse utilization studies in Turkey. Impressions gleaned from observation, from interviews, and from responses to the 1964 study of nursing suggest that a substantial number of nurses are being used for activities other than nursing. Responses to our nursing survey indicated, however, that only one percent of employed graduates of Turkish nursing schools fill patently non-nursing positions. For instance, one was a pharmacy technician while another was a chief *saglik memuru*.

Lack of discrimination in assigning nurses according to their level of preparation leads almost inevitably to inefficient use. The cloudy relationship between nurses and *saglik memurus* leads to individuals being appointed to positions for which they were not prepared. Because physicians greatly outnumber nurses, they personally assume responsibility for elements of patient care that would be better done by nurses. Instances of this are particularly evident in certain teaching and research hospitals connected with the older medical schools where registered nurses are fewer in relation to the number of beds than in most service hospitals. Residents, medical students, and auxiliary nursing personnel perform most of the nursing care. Although this system reduces the budget allocation required for nurses, it has two disadvantages. Patients are likely to receive less skilled nursing care. Doctors learn little of the value and scope of proper nursing because they work only with poorly trained auxiliaries. One professor in a chest disease hospital connected with a medical school regretted the lack of registered nurses in his hospital. Yet when he was asked how he would use one on his service, he quickly replied "as a laboratory technician in my research work."

Lack of clearly defined lines of authority for nursing care creates administrative difficulties. For example, according to written regulations, nurses are required to do whatever the doctor tells them. This directive sounds clear enough. But in most government hospitals many important decisions concerning patient care are left to the few registered nurses or their less qualified substitutes. They are often the only trained personnel covering the wards for eighteen hours through the afternoon and night because the large medical staff withdraws to its private medical practices after 2:00 P.M.

A major hindrance to administrative reform is the widespread practice in Turkey of permitting positions budgeted for one type of personnel to be used for another, even though the functions might be quite different and the institutions widely separated. For example, in 1964, a large urban teaching health center had no public health nurses because the five budgeted positions for public health nurses were being used for midwives in another institution. The lack of nurse teachers in health schools and health colleges is due in large part to this flexible substitution of budgeted positions.

CONDITIONS OF WORK

Working conditions for nurses are particularly unfavorable in Turkey. Long hours of work and uncertain responsibilities are seldom compensated for by appropriate salaries and living arrangements. Average weekly working hours for most active nurses, as reported in the 1964 nursing study, were longer than the usual 44-hour week expected of most other government employees. Over 73 percent of 420 respondents reported that they worked an average of 45 or more hours per week. Over 30 percent worked more than 60 hours per week, and over 13 percent averaged over 72 hours per week.

A majority of active nurses received net salaries of less than $80 per month. Sixty-five percent of 452 respondents received less than 700 TL ($78) per month. More than half of these (37 percent of respondents) received less than 500 TL ($56). Only about one percent of employed nurses received 1,500 TL ($167) or more per month, despite the fact that over 16 percent were directors of nursing in hospitals or in nursing schools. Although most nurses working in hospitals receive free accommodation and meals, equivalent living allowances are not provided for hospital nurses who live at home or for nurses working in public health programs, except in the nationalized health services. The five to eight years compulsory service required of nurses who graduate from Ministry of Health training programs may in the future become a serious impediment to satisfactory recruitment.

For practical planning purposes it was desirable to get more precise information on the specific working conditions that nurses would consider acceptable. Their preferences were indicated by their frank responses in the 1964 survey. Both active and inactive nurses were asked to select one of six employment plans.

The first three plans specified that the nurse could choose her place of work but other variables were limited to the following combinations of working hours and salary:

Plan A. Twenty hours duty per week with one-half the usual salary.

Plan B. Forty hours duty per week with the usual salary.

Plan C. Voluntary work without pay.

The next three plans allowed no choice in the place to which the nurse would be assigned to work and specified the following alternatives:

Plan D. Indefinite hours of duty with double the usual salary.
Plan E. Present working hours with somewhat higher pay.
Plan F. Eight-hour shifts, six days per week, at the usual salary for day duty and 20 percent additional for evening and night duty.

For those who were not in favor of any of these alternatives two additional responses were in the questionnaire. "None of the above conditions are suitable to me," or "not willing to work as a nurse in Turkey under any conditions."

Preferences of 619 respondents are shown in Table 4–9. Most active nurses selected the "no choice of place" option and this group were equally divided between Plans E and F involving higher salary with the same working hours or a clear limitation of working hours with extra pay only for overtime. Those active nurses who wanted to "choose place of work" favored Plan B for a "forty-hour week at present pay scales." In contrast, inactive nurses expressed greatest interest in being allowed to choose their place of work, a response certainly related to their family obligations. They also showed a preference for regular working hours.

TABLE 4–9. NURSES' PREFERENCES IN WORKING CONDITIONS RELATED TO ACTIVITY STATUS

Options	% Active (N = 499)	% Inactive (N = 157)
Place of her own choice with:	20.6	35.0
Plan A—20-hour duty at ½ present pay scales	(0.8)	(7.6)
Plan B—40-hour duty at present pay scales	(18.8)	(18.5)
Plan C—Volunteer work	(1.0)	(8.9)
No choice of place with:	51.6	15.9
Plan D—Indefinite hours at double present salary	(1.2)	—
Plan E—Present working hours with higher pay	(24.7)	(10.2)
Plan F—8-hour shifts, 6 days per week with extra		
pay for evening and night duties	(25.7)	(5.7)
None of the above plans	16.6	26.1
Not willing to work in Turkey	5.2	18.5
No answer	6.0	4.5
Total	100.0	100.0

Although the responses to this question do not allow us to rank the various aspects of working conditions in the order of their importance to nurses, they do give reactions to practical alternatives which are useful guides to policy determination.

More than one-fourth of the respondents stated that none of the options presented was suitable or that they would not consider working as a nurse in Turkey under any conditions. In order to identify the other conditions which nurses see as unfavorable to the profession, respondents were asked to specify problems they considered more pertinent than the plans listed. The 61 percent who responded ranked as most important: "suitable housing " and "better attitudes of doctors." These were followed by "respect shown by auxiliaries," "clear definition of duties," and "title of nurse reserved for graduate."

LOSS AND RETURN OF ACTIVE NURSES

Excessive speculation without factual information about nurses leaving Turkey tends to exaggerate the numbers. The real issue is that it is usually the most competent and best educated nurses who leave. Equally important was the probability that many of those leaving the country do not return to active nursing in Turkey. Of the 377 nurses working in Turkey who answered the question about going abroad, 18 percent indicated that they planned to go abroad in twelve months. Also out of 499 respondents actively nursing in Turkey, 25 percent said they planned to leave nursing within the year and 18 percent more said they might. Balancing all responses, the most conservative estimate extrapolated to the total supply of active nurses, is that about 570 (34%) of the 1683 nurses estimated to be active in the first half of 1964 would leave nursing in Turkey within a year. These could be replaced only in part by an estimated 318 nurses who were inactive, including those abroad. Although the remaining gap could be filled by the 1964 graduates, the size of the real increment for the year would be only about 1 percent.

TRENDS IN NURSE SUPPLY

Over a period of thirty-eight years the annual increment of active nurses has been small but gradually increasing. Table 4–10 lists the number of graduates according to time periods coinciding with important stages in the development of nursing education in Turkey. From 1927 to 1941, the one existing school graduated an average of 23 nurses per year. The increased number of schools and health colleges has brought the annual number of graduates to an average of 197. Population growth has canceled out part of the expected improvement in that the ratio of population to nurses has gone from 37,912 people per active nurse in 1927 to 16,171 per active nurse in 1964. Hence while the number of nurses has increased by eight times, the nurse/population ratio has decreased by only half. Table 4–10 also shows that the number of graduates has been increasing at a slower rate than the number of nursing schools, obviously due to smaller graduating classes per school.

TABLE 4–10. NUMBER OF PROFESSIONAL NURSE GRADUATES AND ESTIMATES OF CUMULATIVE NUMBER ACTIVE IN TURKEY AND INCREMENTS BY TIME PERIODS, 1927–64

Year	Number of schools graduating students during period	Graduates		(Active in Turkey (Est.)	
		Total number	Yearly average	Cumulative no. at end of period	Average annual increment
1927–41	1	344	23	228	15
1942–4	2	149	50	341	38
1945–54	6	804	80	902	56
1955–8	10	481	120	1,167	66
1959–64	12	1,185	197	1,852	121

Table 4–11 shows that there were sufficient applicants for nurse training since acceptance rates for all schools were below 50 percent. The low admission rates indicate either that many unqualified candidates are applying or that student enrollment could in fact be increased. The cost of doubling enrollment in the present schools would be far less than the capital investment required to open new schools. Even though the Ministry of Health has increased the number of schools which offer basic nursing, the enrollment of *female* students is very small. During 1964–5, the nine new health colleges sponsored by the Ministry of Health had a total enrollment of 794, of which only 9 percent were females.

The two higher schools of nursing recently established by the Ministry of Health will not significantly increase the numbers of nurses. Their graduates are expected to provide leadership in nursing education and administrative services. However, present policies in these schools discourage recruitment. Lack of satisfactory

TABLE 4–11. TOTAL NUMBER OF ACADEMICALLY QUALIFIED APPLICANTS AND
PROPORTION ADMITTED TO LYCEE-LEVEL NURSING SCHOOLS AND HEALTH COLLEGES
(1962–63)

Type of school	Number of institutions	Total number of applicants	Admitted		% Female students
			No.	%	
Sponsored by voluntary agencies	3	266	118	44.4	100
Health colleges for nurse-midwifery	2	231	78	33.8	100
Health colleges for nurses	3	383	99	25.8	100
Health colleges for both female nurses & *saglik memurus*	5	1,908	218	11.4	26
Yenisehir Health College, Ankara	1	2,220	100	8.2	13
Total	14[a]	4,008	613	15.3	

[a] Nine additional schools were opened in the latter part of 1963. No information
was obtained from these schools.

boarding facilities at the Florence Nightingale College of Nursing
keeps the enrollment low. At Gevher Nesibe Health Institute the
capacity is limited and *saglik memurus* are given preference (or at
least equal opportunity) in admissions. Another policy of the Ministry of Health which will also limit recruitment is the requirement
that graduates of the Florence Nightingale College of Nursing serve
eight years while other higher schools of nursing have much less or
no compulsory service. Since compulsory service interferes with the
natural inclination for young women to marry and start their
families, many potential recruits would probably avoid committing
themselves for twelve continuous years of employment in nursing.

COST OF NURSING EDUCATION

Definitive cost studies of nursing education are urgently needed.
The total expenditure for nursing education has probably increased
markedly with doubling of the number of lycee-level schools and
four new higher nursing schools since 1961. Extending the teaching
programs from three to four years adds about 25 percent to the
cost of each graduate. In addition, the inclusion of more courses in
general education requires additional teachers for these subjects.

Particularly difficult to estimate is the unit cost of educating a nurse. On the basis of information supplied by two lycee-level schools of nursing sponsored by voluntary agencies the costs range from about 28,000 TL ($3,000) to 42,000 TL ($4,700) per nurse graduate for clearly determinable expenditures. In these calculations it was assumed that student services to hospitals balanced the cost of providing this part of the education.

The difficulty of obtaining valid and comparable cost figures for all lycee-level schools of nursing is illustrated by differences in their administrative organization. Seven colleges have only day students who are not provided with pocket money or living allowances, one school has both day students and boarders, and the other colleges have only boarders. Ratios of full-time nurse teaching staff to students vary from 1/15 to 1/101, and total enrollments range from 32 to 228. Other problems include varying systems of accounting for expenditures, estimating the value of services provided to a hospital by students and staff in relation to the hospital's cost in providing clinical experience, separating out general operating costs, and establishing standard procedures for amortization of investments in buildings and permanent equipment.

SUMMARY AND IMPLICATIONS

The lack of adequately trained nursing personnel in Turkey has severely hampered improvement of urban health services and it is certain to interfere with expansion of rural programs. The problem of over-all shortage is compounded by imbalances in utilization of nurses. In 1964, the ratio of registered nurses to population was estimated to be only 5.5 per 100,000, an extremely unfavorable index compared with many developed countries. Regional distributions varied widely, going as low as one nurse for over 87,000 people in southeastern Anatolia. Nurses, even more than doctors and hospital beds, were concentrated in the three metropolitan areas. The most dramatic evidence of imbalance is that there were about five doctors for every registered nurse.

Two major constraints have limited the increase in active supply: slow expansion in the production of new nurses and a serious gap between leakage from and retrieval to active professional work. In almost four decades the number of nursing schools increased 12-fold, while the average number of female nurses graduating annually increased only 8-fold and the handful of active nurses per 100,000 population was only doubled. This suggests that there is poor utilization of schools and also that there are significant deterrents to remaining active in nursing in Turkey. Even though survey findings show that marriage and child rearing are the main reasons for leaving active nursing, these could be temporary losses. Much more important are the permanent losses due to unsatisfactory working conditions and low prestige, which make the profession unattractive to potential returnees and suitable recruits.

Although three main levels (university, lycee, middle school) of trained nursing personnel exist, there is little or no distinction in functions between the categories. Trained nurses' aides and registered nurses are used interchangeably even for skilled nursing care and administration of nursing services. A cloudy relationship between nurses and the more numerous *saglik memurus* favors advancement of the men into teaching and administrative positions in nursing even though their training and experience are in quite different activities. A substantial number of registered nurses are used for activities other than nursing, while much of the direct care of patients is provided by untrained patient helpers. Furthermore, the custom of freeing doctors for private practice after 2:00 P.M. leaves the few nurses in many hospitals with heavy responsibilities for decisions regarding patient care. Meanwhile, ironically, upper level budgeted nursing positions which would attract well-prepared nurses are often used for doctors.

Policies concerning nurses' functions, standards of education, qualifications for registration and eventual appointment are determined largely by the Ministry of Health. Most decisions are made, however, by doctors while nurses in the Bureau of Nursing and in other nursing groups have little opportunity to guide policies concerned with nursing.

It is unlikely that gradual changes with partial measures and a piecemeal approach will correct the serious deficiencies of nursing in Turkey. In order to develop an adequate supply of professional and middle level nurses in terms of numbers and preparation, radical changes are necessary simultaneously in present education, utilization, and working conditions of nurses.

The first need is for a rationally planned system of nursing. A three-level system for basic nursing services has been recommended by the WHO Expert Committee on Nursing.[5]

1. A fully prepared (professional level) nurse with broadly based education for work in a wide variety of situations demanding a high quality of judgment and decision.

2. A middle level nurse with training for providing preventive and curative care to individuals and groups, with emphasis on technical rather than general competence.

3. An aide who is prepared through short technical training courses to carry out specific tasks of limited scope.

This system should encompass men as well as women, also mid-wifery, psychiatry and public health as well as general nursing in hospitals. Once the necessary categories have been defined, the ratios or mix of nursing personnel required must vary according to the kinds of services to be provided and according to the level of education available in the manpower pool of the country.

Male nurses are needed because they are more effective than women in certain kinds of curative and preventive nursing work such as care of male patients with mental illness and V.D., or for rural health work in remote areas where living and travel may be too arduous for female public health nurses. Although male nurses are successfully included in the nursing systems of many countries, in Turkey a different arrangement might work more effectively for the development of comprehensive nursing services. Considering the cultural climate of Turkey it might be best to maintain the present separate, all-male *saglik memuru* system of education and services, including special types of nursing. In any event, a clear decision needs to be made on how male nurses will be fitted into Turkey's nursing system. Regardless of what decision is made about the location of saglik memurus in relation to the system, it is imperative that those responsible for nursing care of patients be controlled by the same regulations for education and practice that apply to nurses.

An essential component of a national nursing system is effective utilization of personnel. For this, careful studies of patient care are needed in Turkey to define roles, responsibilities and patterns of staffing of health personnel in a variety of situations. The new national health services provide an important starting place for such studies because of the large investment, many uncertainties and tremendous opportunities for developing unique approaches for effective use of health manpower.

The new nursing system must have a new set of Turkish designations for nursing personnel. It would probably be best to discard the present term for nurse, "hemsire," altogether. This word carries an age-old stigma of low prestige. It cannot be used for men in nursing. It has been used so loosely for trained and untrained personnel alike that it prevents the identification of a recognized professional group. Whatever names are substituted they should reflect real differences in education and responsibilities for the respective categories.

Exceptionally favorable working conditions are essential for trained nursing personnel because theirs is hardship work. Besides having to bear the traditional stigma attached to nursing and emotional strain arising from care of the sick, nurses are prevented from supplementing their salaries through the sorts of private work customarily permitted teachers, doctors and other professionals. These difficulties might be counterbalanced and nursing made more attractive if preferential service policies were provided for nurses. Instead of paying nurses only according to the usual salary scales for government employees based on years of education and service, nurses' salaries could be supplemented with compensatory allowances for difficult work. Such a policy succeeded in attracting health personnel to work in remote areas of the nationalized health services.

Along with special financial incentives, radical departures from the usual regulations regarding conditions of work for government employees could increase recruitment into nursing as well as encourage married nurses to continue active in nursing. In creating unusually favorable working conditions for nurses the focus should be on relieving major deterrents to recruitment and continuing employment. Specifically we refer to the conditions which interfere with a woman's natural inclination toward marriage and child rearing, such as too long a period of compulsory service following a long period of training, working hours which are incompatible with responsibilities at home, living arrangements for staff in hospitals. In order to maintain an adequate nurse supply in competition with other occupational groups it will be necessary to drastically reduce the usual compulsory service requirements, to provide for a 40-hour week with 8-hour shifts, or for part-time work, and to grant housing allowances in lieu of living accommodation in hospitals or other institutions. A precedent for preferential working conditions has already been set in the case of the 34-hour work week for government doctors. Furthermore, provision of preferential working conditions for nurses will not be too high a price to pay if concern about the shortage of nurses is real.

Budgeted positions in nursing—especially high-level ones for teachers, supervisors, and administrators—should be restricted to those with appropriate nursing qualifications. This would require a radical departure from the longstanding and widespread administrative practice in Turkish government services in which positions are "borrowed" from one type of service or institution in order to provide staff for another. However, when nurses know that opportunities for advancement are open to them on the basis of qualifications they are more likely to work for better preparation and performance in nursing.

Finally, a basic change in attitude is fundamental. In planning for education, utilization and compensation of nurses at the professional level, policy makers must think in terms of a group which will be on a par with other professional groups in Turkish society. Here as in other advancing societies a respected leadership group is essential for the development of a nurse supply, adequate in quantity and quality to meeting the growing demand for services.

Concomitantly, professional nurses in Turkey must think beyond the narrow boundaries of a "closed shop" focussed on enhancing their own prestige and constructing a nursing hierarchy. Their real concern should be to develop an effective nursing system through which trained nursing personnel with varied skills and different levels of responsibility provide a broad range of nursing and midwifery services inside and outside hospitals, in rural as well as urban communities.

Note: The foregoing chapter was prepared with special reference to the following sources:

Central Treaty Organization, Conference on Nursing Education, Teheran, Iran, April 14–25, 1964.
Report submitted by the Turkish Nurses Association to the Ministry of Health, May 15, 1963. Published in the *Journal of the Turkish Nurses Association*, Bozak Press, Istanbul, 1964.
Progress reports on projects and field visits made by WHO staff. (Unpublished.)

REFERENCES

1 Shirley Epir, "Profile of the Turkish Nurse," in *Role Image and Professional Opportunities for Nurses in Turkey*. A study conducted by Institute of Research and Service in Nursing Education (Teachers College, Columbia University, March, 1964). (Unpublished.)

2. *Report of Educational Survey Preliminary to Establishment of the Florence Nightingale Higher Educational Program for Nursing* (Teachers College, Columbia University, New York, N.Y., October 31, 1959–January 19, 1960).
3. Alice M. Forman, *A Study of Career Patterns of Turkish Nurses.* Unpublished paper. Analysis of data for this study was supported, in part, by the Faculty Research Development Program Grant (PHS NU00154).
4. Surgeon General's Group on Nursing, *Toward Quality in Nursing: Needs and Goals* (Washington; USPHS, 1963), p. 20.
5. World Health Organization Expert Committee on Nursing. Fifth Report, WHO Technical Report Series No. 347. Geneva, 1966, pp. 11–13.

5

SUPPLY OF OTHER TRAINED HEALTH PERSONNEL

Turkey's shortage of all categories of health personnel is both quantitative and qualitative. The ratio of paramedical and auxiliary health personnel per doctor is 2:1. In the United States the figure is more than 10:1. The most acute manpower problem, however, is maldistribution and misuse. This chapter briefly describes all trained health personnel, other than doctors and nurses, who contribute to the health services of Turkey.

DENTISTS: A PROBLEM OF DISTRIBUTION

No specific census or detailed survey was undertaken to study dental manpower. Existing information was analyzed and the basic problems are so evident that they can be clearly stated.

Historical Information

Turkey's first dental school was established in Istanbul in 1909. The period of training was three years and the prerequisite was middle school, up until 1925 when the entrance level was raised to lycee. In 1933 the length of training was extended to four years. In 1963 three new dental schools were established which included a private school in Istanbul and two schools in Ankara, one attached to the Ankara Medical School and one attached to Hacettepe Medical Center.

Education

Dental training requires four years in the two Istanbul dental schools and five years in the two Ankara schools. Istanbul Dental

163

School produced 2,438 graduates between 1923 and 1964. Table 5–1 shows total students at all dental schools during the 1964–5 academic year. Approximately 150 dentists per year are graduated from the Istanbul school. When the three other schools begin to produce graduates, the number could reach 350.

TABLE 5–1. NUMBER OF STUDENTS ATTENDING DENTAL SCHOOLS DURING 1964–5

Name of school	No. of students
Istanbul University Dental School	564
Private dental school	393
Ankara Dental School	53
Hacettepe Dental School	59
Total	1,069

Duties, Responsibilities, and Salary

As in most countries, dentists extract teeth, fill cavities, make bridges, and treat all diseases of the teeth and gingiva. Very little attention is given to preventive work. Foreign dentists are not permitted to practice in Turkey. The salary for dentists who work as government employees starts at 607.50 TL ($67.50) per month, with an increase to 675 TL ($75) in two years and a promotion every three years after that. The same pay scale applies to dentists working in the nationalized health services, but with additional compensations.

Current Supply of Dentists in Turkey

According to the 1955 census, there were 1,466 dentists living in Turkey, or one dentist for every 16,450 persons. In 1960 the number of dentists was 1,617 or one dentist for every 17,200 inhabitants. The lower ratio shows that general population growth is outpacing the output of dentists. In 1960 there were 1,455 dentists living in localities which had 10,000 or more inhabitants which means that 90 percent of the dentists were serving only 30 percent of the population. At the end of 1963, according to the registry of the Ministry of Health 63 percent of the dentists were living in Ankara, Istanbul, and Izmir provinces which contain 15 percent of the total population.

The number of dentists practicing at the end of 1964 was estimated to be 1,741. Only 76 of them or 4 percent were working for the Ministry of Health and 328 or 19 percent were employed by social insurance institutions or state economic enterprises. This leaves 1,337 or 77 percent in private practice. This finding is in sharp contrast to the relative proportions of doctors, most of whom work at least part-time in public facilities.

Each year an increasing number of dentists leave Turkey to work in foreign countries, especially Switzerland and West Germany. No figures could be obtained to quantify this loss.

Although there is no recognized training program for dental technicians, in both rural areas and cities there are individuals who provide some dental services, mostly learned informally while working in dentists' offices. Preparation of dentures as prescribed by dentists is the only work they are officially permitted to do. But most of them actually have an active private practice which includes extractions, filling cavities, and making bridges. In villages and towns these substitute dentists are the main source of dental services.

PHARMACISTS: MOSTLY PRIVATE PRACTITIONERS

In the delivery of medical care, pharmacists have the intrinsic importance of being the final agent in dispensing much of the treatment received by patients. This important role is not reflected in the attention given to them in this study. Only a brief analysis of already available information was attempted because detailed data-gathering would have required the sort of elaborate tracking mechanisms which were developed for nurses and doctors. Since pharmacists have a rather traditional preparation, are almost entirely urban in their location, and are almost exclusively in private practice, this cursory survey was considered sufficient.

Historical Information

Formal education of pharmacists in Turkey began in 1839 with the establishment of a "pharmacy class" at the Istanbul Medical School providing three years' training for army pharmacists. In 1867 civilian training was begun and a pharmacy department was established which eventually became a separate school with a four-year course. At present there are three Turkish pharmacy schools, one attached to Istanbul University, one to Ankara University, and one a private school in Istanbul.

Training

A lycee diploma is required for admission to pharmacy school. The school in Ankara had its first graduating class in 1965, and the private school will produce its first graduates in 1968.

The number of graduates from the Istanbul Pharmacy School between 1923 and 1963 was 2,009, with an average of 50 graduates per year. In recent years they have exceeded 100 per year and the total number of graduates could increase to 200 as the new schools become fully operational.

Duties, Responsibilities, and Salary

The pharmacist prepares and dispenses drugs. He may operate a pharmacy, an apothecary, a drug wholesale house, or a drug production laboratory. Foreign pharmacists are allowed to practice in Turkey. The salary of a pharmacist employed by the Ministry of Health is the same as that of a dentist, 607.50 TL ($67.50) per month to start.

Current Supply of Pharmacists in Turkey

According to the 1960 census there were 1,675 pharmacists living in Turkey, or one pharmacist for every 16,600 persons. The number living in localities which had 10,000 or more inhabitants was 1,464, which means that 87 percent of the pharmacists were serving only 30 percent of the total population. At the end of 1963, according to the Ministry of Health, 59 percent were living in the three most developed provinces, Ankara, Istanbul, and Izmir.

The number of pharmacists practicing at the end of 1964 was estimated to be 1,749, of whom 1,454 or 83 percent were in private practice. As in many countries, this private practice really means that they undertake total responsibility for the diagnosis and treatment of patients. About 15 percent were working for social insurance institutions or for state economic enterprises. Only 2 percent were with the Ministry of Health.

The question arises as to who dispenses drugs in the 252 hospitals attached to the Ministry of Health. There are no trained technicians to serve as assistant pharmacists in Turkey as there are in some countries. Consequently, most of this work is done by laymen who receive only on-the-job training.

Looking to the future, additions to supply will barely keep up with population increase. The need of the private sector and urban areas will continue to be met. The public sector, however, will continue to have a major deficiency in this important service unless a deliberate effort is made to provide either fully trained or auxiliary pharmacists for public institutions.

THE *SAGLIK MEMURU*: AN ALL-PURPOSE HEALTH TECHNICIAN

Anyone interested in Turkish health manpower quickly becomes acquainted with a multipurpose health worker known as the *saglik memuru*. This individual is "everything and nothing" since he receives rudimentary preparation for many jobs in the health field but very little intensive training and education in any aspect of medical technology. He is a veritable chameleon in his health work, filling gaps in health services from the basic tasks of sanitarians, laboratory technicians, and nurses to performing the duties of a medical officer of health. In rural areas the *saglik memuru* may unofficially serve as a near-doctor or *feldsher*. The following titles are given to the *saglik memuru:* health officer, health technician, sanitarian, and male nurse. The duties and responsibilities of the *saglik memuru* are obviously not clearly defined and many types of assistant health personnel with various educational backgrounds and functions have the title of *saglik memuru*.

Throughout this volume there is an obvious lack of information about manpower for the critically important health needs in sanitation. The little sanitation work that is done is the responsibility of *saglik memurus*.

Historical Information

The *saglik memuru* has had a checkered history. The first school for their training was established in Istanbul in 1910 by Professor Omer of the Istanbul Medical School. Boys and girls who had completed middle school were accepted for two years' training. In 1919 this school was closed because of a plan to establish a school for village doctors.

In 1924, three schools for *saglik memurus*, in Istanbul, Corum, and Sivas, were established by the Ministry of Health. These schools accepted male students after middle school. After many shifts and alterations, all other schools were combined with a school in Ankara in 1954 and training was extended to three years. A student who had dropped out of medical school after completing six semesters or who had graduated from an army or navy noncommissioned health officer's school was accepted as a *saglik memuru* by the Ministry of Health. In 1961 another major reorganization led to the development of the health colleges which took over and greatly expanded the training of *saglik memurus*.

The total number of graduates from all schools for *saglik memurus* between the years 1925 and 1961 was 2,636 with the average annual number of graduates increasing steadily from 22 per year to over 400 in 1961.

The village *saglik memuru* is a special subcategory of personnel who have contributed importantly to rural health services. They were trained first as an off-shoot of the general program of rural development that started some twenty-five years ago. In institutes established mainly for training village school teachers, a special curriculum was set up for *saglik memurus*. Mostly rural candidates with a primary-school education were accepted and given five years' training.

More than 3,000 village *saglik memurus* were trained and stationed in scattered villages. The government then discontinued the training program and the whole village institute system was abandoned in 1954. This decision is now recognized to have been a mistake because of the growing manpower gap in providing trained personnel for the villages. The rural situation became even more acute after a law was passed which allowed village *saglik memurus* to work in towns and cities after they had completed six years of service in villages and passed a special six-month course.

Present Training

The Ministry of Health decided in 1961 to combine all schools of nursing, midwifery, and *saglik memurus* attached to the Ministry of Health into new institutions called health colleges. The period of training was extended from three to four years with all students studying more or less the same subjects during the first three years and specializing during the fourth. The fields of specialization are: male nursing (*saglik memurus*), female nursing, midwifery, environmental sanitation, laboratory technician, and X-ray technician. At present there are fourteen health colleges in Turkey. Two of them accept only male students, six accept only female students, and the others are co-educational. In the 1964–5 academic year there were 1,792 male students attending these colleges, many of whom will become *saglik memurus*.

The curriculum includes professional and cultural courses and practical work in local health institutions. Anatomy, physiology, preventive medicine and public health, bacteriology, surgery, internal medicine, infectious and social diseases, maternal and child health, environmental health, public health administration, health education, and mental health are taught. Cultural lessons, which make up one third of the curriculum are: Turkish language, history, geography, foreign language, physical education, national defense, and general science.

Further Training Possibilities

A saglik memuru is eligible for further training at Gevher Nesibe Institute providing that he has had three years of service and that he passes the entrance examination. Gevher Nesibe offers three years of post-basic education. Graduates are assigned as teachers and administrators in health colleges and health schools or they may be assigned administrative posts in the health services.

Duties and Responsibilities

At the present time there are no definite laws governing the saglik memuru. An official memorandum was published more than twenty-five years ago which states some of their functions. The usual duties include regular monthly visits to villages for improvement of sanitary conditions, investigation of outbreaks of communicable diseases, medical examination of teachers and students in villages, immunization against smallpox and other diseases, preparation of statistical tables and reports for official records, and other miscellaneous preventive and health services. They also serve as statistical clerks, secretaries, and store accountants.

Obviously, the training and education which a *saglik memuru* receives is not adequate for him to meet all these expectations. Because of such frustrations, many of these potentially important health personnel have left government service to work in private business as clerks.

In an effort to attract *saglik memurus* to return to health work, their duties have been made more specific. In the 1963 regulations for nationalization of health services, the *saglik memuru* was made responsible for health education, environmental sanitation, school health, vaccination, first aid, patient care and follow-up in villages—all under the direction of the health unit doctor. He also supervises the work of village midwives, malaria surveillance agents, and trachoma drug applicators.

Current Supply

According to the 1955 census there were 5,557 *saglik memurus* in Turkey. This figure included those with and without diplomas as well as the village *saglik memurus*. Of these 2,279 (41 percent) were living in localities which had 10,000 or more inhabitants while 3,278 (59 percent) were living in more rural localities. It was impossible to get any data from the 1960 census because *saglik memurus* were combined with malaria surveillance agents and other male health workers.

The following figures were obtained from the *Saglik Memurus'* Association. At the beginning of 1964 the number of *saglik memurus* on their rolls was: 2,350 with diplomas; 3,100 village *saglik memurus*, and 310 without diplomas—totaling 5,760. According to Ministry of Health data there were 5,996 *saglik memurus* in Turkey at the end of 1964 (Table 5–2), the large majority being employed by the government.

TABLE 5–2. NUMBER OF *Saglik Memurus* ACCORDING TO PLACE OF EMPLOYMENT (AT THE END OF 1964)

Place of employment	Type of *saglik memuru*	No.
Ministry of Health	*Saglik memuru*	2,079
Ministry of Health	Village *saglik memuru*	1,409
Municipality & local government	*Saglik memuru*	213
Municipality & local government	Village *saglik memuru*	8
Private office	*Saglik memuru*	123
Other places	*Saglik memuru* and village *saglik memuru*	2,125
Not working	*Saglik memuru*	39
Total		5,996

Process of Assignment, Salary, and Promotion

The three top graduates of each school are assigned to the type of work and areas for which they apply and the remainder draw lots. Anyone who requests an assignment in the nationalized health services must sign a three-year contract.

Saglik memurus are ranked as lycee graduates on the pay scale. The government scale starts at 472.50 TL ($52.50) per month with increments every three years to a maximum of 2,025.00 TL ($225.00) after thirty years. However, promotions are not automatic since they depend on the availability of budgeted positions. Those *saglik memurus* who work in nationalized health services receive traveling expenses and special compensations for the place of work according to degree of deprivation in particular geographical areas. With these compensations a *saglik memuru* may make a beginning salary of 1,272.50 TL ($141) per month.

THE MIDWIFE: AN ESSENTIAL SERVICE WHICH ACTUALLY REACHES THE RURAL AREAS

In all countries and throughout history some individuals have been recognized to have special skills in helping pregnant women in labor. In most societies an early synthesis of knowledge led to formal transmission of skills and the midwife had a systematized social role. Where societies were sufficiently affluent, doctors themselves took responsibility for deliveries under the more dignified title of obstetrics. Most babies around the world are delivered not by doctors but by trained or untrained women practicing midwifery. Their titles are as numerous as their training and experience is diverse.

There are three types of trained midwives in Turkey: the nurse midwife, the urban midwife, and the rural midwife. The *ebe anne* or traditional birth attendant will not be included in this chapter because she receives no formal training and is therefore considered later with traditional health workers.

Particularly important in the transition to systematically organized modern midwifery is an emphasis on prevention. Antenatal and postnatal services are provided mainly through maternal and child health clinics. These clinics also provide parallel programs concerned with infant mortality and morbidity.

Rapid expansion of family-planning services has been officially recognized as a major new obligation of government health services in Turkey. The rapid population growth directly jeopardizes both health and economic development. Although the details of the new national program have not yet been defined, it is clear that midwives will fill an important role.

Historical Information

The first organized effort to train midwives in Turkey was in 1842 when an Italian doctor started a two-year midwifery school in Istanbul. In 1890 Professor Omer opened a school which accepted primary-school graduates for midwifery training. This school was affiliated with the Istanbul University Medical School in 1910. In 1924 entrance requirements were changed to middle-school graduates.

In 1937 rural midwifery training was started when two village-midwifery schools were opened by the Ministry of Health. Admission was limited to girls who had completed primary school and were fifteen to eighteen years of age. In 1961, the name Village Midwifery School was changed to Health School and many new schools were opened. The length of study was extended from one year to three years.

The Ministry of Health opened its first urban midwifery school in 1953 at the Ankara Maternity Hospital. It later became a nurse-midwife school and the length of training was extended to four years. In 1961, all schools for nurse-midwives which were operated by the Ministry of Health were incorporated into the health colleges. The Ankara Nurse-Midwives School became the Ankara Maternity Hospital Health College, and Zeynep Kamil Health College in Istanbul was devoted to midwifery training.

Due to the almost constant changes which have taken place in midwifery training during the past twenty years, there is great variation from one age bracket of midwives to another in the amount of schooling, the curriculum, and especially the amount of practical training. The differences between rural and urban midwives are particularly marked.

The Village Midwife

The delivery of a baby in most of rural Turkey is still attended by an *ebe anne* (traditional birth attendant), a member of the family, a friend or a neighbor. The Ministry of Health has tried to expand the village midwifery program but has only made a beginning. Village midwives are trained at the twenty-five health schools established by the Ministry of Health. The course of studies is three years, with admission after five years of preliminary schooling. Although the curriculum emphasizes supervised practical experience in midwifery, instruction in general nursing, child health, and cultural subjects is included. The curriculum also covers basic sciences and language, preventive and curative medicine, infectious and social diseases, and maternal and child health. Most of these schools are connected with maternity hospitals. The number of students attending these schools in 1964 was 1,587. If present expectations are met, there will be about 500 graduates per year.

From 1938 to 1964 there were 4,633 graduates from all the village midwifery schools and health schools.

Lack of qualified teaching staff is perhaps the most urgent problem for the health schools. In 1964, in all of the health schools there were only three midwives and twenty-five nurses working as full-time professional teachers and twenty-five part-time doctors acting as directors. This is a ratio of 61 students per full-time nurse and per part-time doctor and 529 students per midwife.

Village midwives earn 405 TL ($45) per month as a beginning salary. After three years they are raised to 472.50 TL ($52.50) per month, which is the starting salary of urban midwives. Every three years thereafter they are promoted. Those who work in nationalized health services get additional compensations including housing.

The duties and responsibilities of the village midwife include conducting deliveries, making regular visits to homes where there are pregnant women or newborn babies, providing antenatal and post-partum services, collecting statistical information on births and deaths, and follow-up of patients at home as ordered by the health center doctor.

Village midwives who have completed a minimum of six years of successful work in villages may take a six-month practical course in a maternity hospital. Then after passing an examination, they are permitted to practice in towns and cities, either privately or in institutions.

The number of village midwives actively working at the end of 1964 was 3,104, according to the Ministry of Health, which means that 66 percent of the graduates were known to be actually working. We could not obtain information on whether the remaining village midwives were working privately, employed outside the usual governmental organizations, or unemployed.

As indicated in Table 5–3, in addition to the 2,534 village midwives employed by the Ministry in villages, there were 561 village midwives who had made the transition to urban areas. Of these, 279 (9 percent) were employed by the municipalities and local authorities in urban maternity hospitals or in dispensaries and 282 were employed directly by the Ministry of Health in urban health centers. Ninety percent of all village midwives employed by the Ministry of Health were actually working in rural areas. In 1964 the ratio of trained midwives to population was only slightly lower in rural areas then in urban areas (1.34/10,000 *vs.* 1.47/10,000). This ratio for midwives is more favorable for the rural population than the ratio for any other type of health personnel.

TABLE 5–3. DISTRIBUTION OF TRAINED MIDWIVES (1964)

Working in	Midwives trained for rural areas	Midwives trained for urban areas	Totals	Population	Ratio of midwives per 10,000 population
Villages	2,534	—	2,534	18,895,084	1.34
Cities and towns	561	1,048	1,609	10,900,000	1.47
Total	3,104	1,048	4,152	29,795,084	

Even so, coverage is far from adequate. Accessibility to trained health personnel is, of course, more difficult in rural areas because of transportation and communication problems. According to a country-wide* sample study in 1963, only 7 percent of deliveries in villages were attended by trained personnel whereas the rate was 31 percent in cities and towns. Perhaps the most relevant issue is that rural midwives are supposed to concentrate on preventive activities. In rural areas midwives probably do, in fact, put most of their effort into prenatal and postnatal care while traditional birth attendants may actually conduct the deliveries.

The crude birth rate in the rural areas is 45.2 per 1,000 population which is considerably higher than the 28 per 1,000† rate of cities and towns. Calculating from the crude birth rate and population figures for the rural area and the number of rural midwives, it is estimated that there are 302 births per rural midwife per year. The number of births that each midwife can attend depends mainly on accessibility and geographical location. Since the rural population is scattered, it is apparent that the present supply of midwives could not possibly be available for all deliveries, even if the village people were to ask for their help.

Only 15 percent‡ of the population in rural areas of Turkey have trained midwives available. Only 10 percent§ of the 35,444 villages

*Population Growth Study in Turkey, conducted by Dr. George W. Angell in 1963.

†Report of the Study of Births and Deaths in a Sample Population in Turkey in 1963, by Kathleen Gales for Ministry of Health, Ankara (unpublished).

‡Source: 1963 Muhtar Survey described in Chapter 6 on indigenous health workers covering 89 percent of 35,444 villages which included 88 percent of the rural population.

§10.1 percent is based on data obtained from the 1963 Muhtar Survey. 10.2 percent is the proportion when official figures of the Ministry of Health are used.

have trained resident midwives. Although these midwives are usually employed by the government and each is expected to be available to women in five or six villages, their delivery services are generally limited to the larger villages where they reside.

Where trained personnel are not easily accessible, the people obviously still rely on untrained persons. Greater use of traditional birth attendants in rural areas is associated with higher infant mortality rates but, of course, other variables associated with village hygienic and nutritional conditions are also partly responsible. In the villages of Turkey the average infant mortality rate is estimated to be approximately 278‖ per thousand live births. This is 43 percent higher than the average rate for metropolitan areas where the infant mortality rate is approximately 158 per thousand live births.

Urban Midwives and Nurse-Midwives

Although there is considerable movement of village midwives to the city, it is not surprising that there is almost no reverse migration. Most of the midwives in urban areas work in hospitals or in Maternal and Child Health Centers. Some have private practices. In the hospitals they are subject to the same regulations and conditions as nurses.

Urban and nurse midwives receive their training at either Ankara Maternity Hospital, Zeynep Kamil in Istanbul, or the Istanbul Midwives School under the Istanbul Medical School. At the two former schools the period of training is four years, while the latter has a two-year course of study. Eight years of preliminary education are required for admission.

According to Ministry of Health statistics, at the end of 1964 there were 1,048 graduates of urban midwifery schools. Of these 283 (27 percent) were in private practice, 542 (52 percent) were in institutions of the state economic enterprises and ministries other than the Ministry of Health, 130 (12.3 percent) worked for municipalities and local governments, and only 93 (8.7 percent) were with the Ministry of Health. More midwives will have to be attracted from other employment to staff the MCH centers where family planning is to be provided, in order to meet the manpower requirement for this new and urgently needed major emphasis.

‖Report of a Study of Births and Deaths in a Sample Population in Turkey in 1963, by Kathleen Gales.

With their more advanced education, the most important functions for which urban midwives can appropriately be used are teaching, administrative and supervisory roles, especially in schools for rural midwives. Rural midwives will be needed in large numbers for the nationalization plan and for the national family-planning program and they cannot be prepared without an increase in the number of teachers in midwifery schools.

THE LACK OF SANITATION PERSONNEL

Among all the health manpower shortages in Turkey the one that stands out most clearly as being totally lacking is sanitation personnel. Nursing shortages are also severe but at least there is official recognition of the deficiency and an effort to correct it. Sanitation is one of the most evident health needs of Turkey by any criterion. As the nationalization program brings health programs to the villages, there will be an immediate need for individuals responsible for improving the physical environment.

In sanitation, the most serious gap is that there is no recognition of the need for systematic provision for clearly defined categories of workers. Until the specified categories are created nothing can be done about training sanitary workers. The *saglik memurus* now include sanitation among the multiple tasks they perform. They receive some training in sanitation and are expected to do most of the work. As has been pointed out, they have been assigned so many tasks that focused attention on one responsibility is impossible.

Sanitary engineers are essentially nonexistent. Urban water supplies and sanitary codes are the responsibility of departments of public works and their civil engineers. Again the shortage of personnel makes for erratic performance.

The simplest procedure administratively would be to have even more sharply defined subspecialization among *saglik memurus*. A large proportion of them should be specially trained for rural sanitation and should then work exclusively on such activities. Ultimately, the best way of providing these services, however, would be to start training a whole new category of sanitarians.

6

TRADITIONAL HEALTH WORKERS IN TURKEY

In every traditional society certain individuals assume responsibility for serving as the repository of the local accumulation of health folklore and clinical skills. In primitive cultures herbs, potions, and body manipulations that have been found to be effective are gradually added to magical and religious practices. Occasional chance discoveries of practical importance are empirically accepted especially when they have dramatic and direct effects. More often religious faith and superstition lead to unquestioning acceptance of many useless practices. Considerable specialization of function marks most indigenous systems, largely because of deliberate efforts to restrict the transmission of healing lore to a small number of initiates.

Traditional health practices are absorbed into or are part and parcel of the whole sociocultural framework of a society. An indigenous practitioner must make sure that his practices comply with community beliefs and values. He is responsible for the local health culture. Popular beliefs about the causation and care of health problems will be dilutions of what the healer believes. Therefore, for the clearest understanding of local beliefs it is often useful to go directly to the aforementioned practitioner.

When professional modern health services are first introduced into a community which has previously met its own health needs, it must be with the realization that the community is not a health care vacuum. If deliveries have been performed by untrained midwives for centuries, the arrival of a trained professional midwife will probably be viewed as a threat by traditional practitioners.

Moreover, the trained professional midwife is often an outsider to the village community with different speech, dress, and manners. She also is usually at the disadvantage of being considerably younger than the traditional midwives. Personal behavior patterns also influence the rate of acceptance by the village community, since villagers are less tolerant of outsiders. Furthermore, many health professionals tend to assume a rather supercilious attitude toward traditional practitioners. Little effort is made to understand local practices or patterns of work and at times the professional seems reluctant to admit that traditional practitioners exist. This, of course, causes resentment.

Since the new nationalization plan stresses the provision of comprehensive health services for rural areas it is especially important to define clearly the role of indigenous health workers.

No studies of the traditional health workers of Turkey have been done. This is partly because all medical practice by indigenous health workers is prohibited by law and it is easier for the government to ignore them. Even cursory review of the law shows the severity of the government's attitude toward this group. Indeed, even free treatment is illegal. The severity of punishment written into the law gives some indication of the relative status of each type of traditional health worker: *Article 25*—Any person without an M.D. diploma who treats patients in any way, even if he does not receive a fee, or who uses the title of "doctor" will be sentenced to one to six months' imprisonment and must pay a fine of 25–500 TL ($3–$55). *Article 41*—Anyone who practices dentistry without a diploma or certificate, even if he does not receive a fee, will be sentenced to fifteen days' to three months' imprisonment. *Article 54*—Anyone who works as a midwife without a diploma or certificate, will be sentenced to seven days' to three months' imprisonment and must pay a fine of 5–50 TL ($.50–$9). *Article 61*—Anyone who works as a circumciser without a certificate or permit will be sentenced to seven days' to one month's imprisonment. *Article 67*—Anyone who works as a nurse or uses the title without a permit must pay a fine of 5–50 TL ($.50–$9).

CATEGORIES OF TRADITIONAL HEALTH WORKERS

Traditional health workers are any individuals who provide health care without having received formal training or a certificate recognized by the government. The various types of traditional workers in Turkey are briefly categorized.

Needleman. His health knowledge may have been derived from military service as a trained medical corpsman, from working in a doctor's office, or from being a janitor in a hospital. Needlemen frequently diagnose, prescribe drugs, and give medical advice in addition to giving injections. They are usually male, over twenty-five years of age, and are often given the title of "doctor" in the village where they practice.

Traditional Birth Attendant or Ebe Anne. These untrained and usually illiterate women conduct deliveries and provide supportive care for maternity cases. They are usually over thirty-five years of age. Through the years, these women tend to accumulate much obstetrical experience but their techniques are based on folklore passed through apprenticeship relationships. They frequently treat sterility, dysmenorrhea, and menorrhagia. They serve one village and work on a fee-for-services basis.

Bone-setters. They are generally male, aged thirty-five or more, and serve more than one village. They reduce dislocations, set fractures, and give advice on the care of these conditions. The knowledge of the bone-setter is usually passed through family relationships. They sometimes also care for animals which have been injured. They charge a fee.

Circumcisers. They are generally male, aged thirty-five or more, and serve more than one village. Circumcision is supposed to be done only by a licensed circumcisers. The indigenous circumcisers, many of whom are gypsies, operate without a license. They charge a fee.

Bloodletters. These practitioners specialize in illnesses caused by "bad blood," i.e., eczema, pain, and cramps. They usually draw blood from the interscapular area or from the site of pain and use a pointed sharp instrument or leeches. They may be either male or female and usually charge for their services. They ordinarily limit their practice to one village.

Lead-pourers. These elderly women, at least fifty years of age, are consulted for illnesses which are believed to be caused by "evil eye." They melt a piece of lead in a pan, pour it into a container of cold water held over the head of the ill person and then try to find the reason for the curse by studying the shape of the lead. Their recommendations rely on magic and suggestion. Sometimes they also give the water into which the lead was poured to the patient to drink. They serve one village. They generally practice on a courtesy basis but occasionally charge a fee.

Tooth-pullers. These practitioners specialize in extractions. They usually have other employment such as barber, blacksmith, or needleman. They are male and charge a fee.

Umbilicus-setters. These practitioners specialize in the treatment of persons who complain of indigestion or abdominal pain. Diagnosis consists of determining the direction of displacement of the umbilicus, often with elaborate measuring and flourishes of magical manipulation. After making a diagnosis they massage the abdomen for five to ten minutes, and then press hard on the umbilicus while pushing it in the appropriate direction. Simultaneously, they say with great authority: "Now your umbilicus is set." They may be either male or female, they serve only their own village, and they sometimes charge fees.

Coccyx-pullers. These practitioners massage and manipulate the lower spine and sacroiliac region for people who have cramps or pain in the back or difficulty walking. They may be either male or female and serve only their own villages. They sometimes charge fees.

Religious teachers. Local religious leaders employ their religious authority to treat patients. They read prayers in Arabic which petition God to heal the patient. They fold Arabic sacred writings into a triangular shape which the patient sews into an amulet and wears about his neck. They also treat abdominal pain and backache by tying a string about the abdomen with a special series of knots. The religious teachers are especially sought out for the treatment of mental illness and epilepsy. They are male and usually over thirty. They serve mainly their own village, unless they achieve fame, and then people travel from other villages to see them. They may or may not charge fees but patients usually make a contribution.

Mystic healers (sorcerers, sacred-house owners). These individuals claim "power" from mystical sources which may be quite varied. Frequently the special power is passed through family lines. The "power" of an individual healer may, however, be derived from a specific healing episode in which a dramatic effect occurred by chance. A healer's reputation may spread over quite an area. They may be either male or female and they normally charge a fee.

SPECIALIZED FUNCTIONS OF TRADITIONAL HEALTH WORKERS

In applying their knowledge to indigenous classifications of symptoms, traditional health workers are "specialists." Roughly they fall into the following classifications:

(a) emergency services or acute illness—Needleman, traditional birth attendant, tooth-puller, bone-setter;
(b) chronic diseases or symptoms—Bloodletter, umbilicus-setter, coccyx-puller, mystic healer, religious teacher;
(c) psychiatric or psychosomatic problems—Religious teacher, lead-pourer, mystic healer.

Many of the indigenous practices of traditional health workers are merely exotic and interesting, but others are distinctly dangerous. Examples picked up in casual conversations with indigenous practitioners are given to illustrate the variety of procedures and treatments used.

Emergency service. A dead spider is placed on a cut or an injury or mud is placed on a bruise; a mixture of ground coffee and yogurt or anything cold is rubbed on a burn; the juice of onion covered with hot ash is put on a paronychia (abscess of the fingernail) and tied in place; a person seriously injured in a fall or accident is covered with the skin of a sheep or goat freshly skinned; in cases of unwanted pregnancy, the woman sits above a grill with hay burning underneath in the belief that the baby will suffocate from the smoke and be forced out of the mother's body; the mother is buried in dung up to the waist if bleeding has not stopped after delivery; because premature births are considered shameful in the case of a new bride, deliveries are prevented in the seventh or eighth month by binding the hips, legs, and abdomen of the pregnant woman even if labor pains have started.

Chronic diseases or symptoms. In treating bone tuberculosis or erythema nodosum, the "healer" calls on mystical power and then touches or spits on the diseased area; in cases of sterility, the woman sits in hot water or a steam bath; the meat of a young dog is fed to a person with tuberculosis; in cases of hemorrhoids, a hole about 3 cm. in diameter is cut in the shell of a live tortoise and the person sits so that the hemorrhoid is in this hole; with malunion or poor alignment of a fracture, an eviscerated fish is placed on the surface of the skin over the fracture site to soften the bone, if the bone is small the fish is kept in place for one day but with larger bones the time is two to three days. When the fish is removed the fracture, supposedly, can be manipulated into proper alignment.

Psychiatric or psychosomatic problems. A person who is always fearful is required to drink the urine of a boy; certain herbs burned over a fire are used for some mental illnesses; a blue bead or an amulet around the neck is worn as protection from the "evil eye"; a psychotic person is tied with rope in a dark place for three days.

INTERRELATIONSHIPS BETWEEN TRADITIONAL HEALTH WORKERS
AND TRAINED HEALTH WORKERS IN RURAL AREAS

The social problems resulting from the introduction of scientific health services into the traditional health culture of rural Turkey have become increasingly evident. Traditional practitioners are locally respected for their knowledge of health lore and are naturally reluctant to surrender the status and prestige they gain from the application of empiric skills.

Village people first learn about scientific medicine through contact with doctors in towns and cities. Stories of dramatic cures circulate and in varying degrees challenge the previously unquestioned authority of traditional practitioners. Some of them incorporate into their own practice a superficial use of the most dramatic and readily learned techniques of scientific medicine. The most important traditional specialists numerically are the needlemen who use the syringe as a symbol of modern medicine because it has acquired a special aura of healing power among the general public.

The first representatives of scientific medicine to personally reside in villages have usually been the *saglik memurus* and trained midwives. Until recently the only doctors working in villages were the medical officers of health who visited periodically to direct rural public health programs.

The lack of planning for health manpower in the past is clearly shown by the frequency with which laws were passed which had no possibility of being implemented. An example is the 1928 law forbidding midwives to deliver babies unless they were certified. If the law had actually been enforced, approximately 300 midwives would have had to deliver each year some 600,000 babies scattered in 35,000 villages. As indicated in the previous section, other articles of the 1928 law made it illegal to practice any type of traditional health work, even though there were no trained workers available to provide minimum services. Thirty-six years later a survey of 90 percent of Turkish villages reported a total of 85,643 indigenous health workers actively in practice, in spite of the law.

An important consideration in manpower planning, then, is that sufficient numbers of trained personnel should be available to be phased in at appropriate stages of any new program. The need is most evident now in Turkey because of the new nationalization plan which has been publicized as an effort to equalize the health benefits provided for rural people. Health functions now performed by traditional workers are supposed to be gradually taken over by trained personnel. The transition will require many years and infinite patience.

To obtain more specific information about village health workers a special study was begun in August, 1963. The primary aim was to determine the geographic distribution of indigenous health workers and their numerical relationship to trained health workers. Additional information was obtained about certain sociological and educational variables that influence their activities. Since there was no direct access to indigenous workers by an existing administrative channel, the most comprehensive approach was to find out from the rural people.

Materials and Methods of Rural Health Workers Survey

The State Institute of Statistics was preparing for a national agricultural census to be asked every village leader (*muhtar*) in Turkey and agreed to include a set of health questions. Because of the co-operation of officials from the statistical institute, data were gathered which would otherwise have been beyond our resources. The State Institute sent instructors to each of the sixty-seven provinces where seminars were held to familiarize agricultural technicians with the questionnaire and to train them in interviewing techniques. Subsequently each agricultural technician invited all village leaders within his area to a central location and completed the questionnaires individually in the *muhtar's* presence.

Since it was impractical to list all categories of indigenous health workers in the questionnaire, only the following were included: needleman, *ebe anne* or traditional birth attendant, circumciser, and bone-setter. Two categories of trained health workers were included for comparison—trained midwives and *saglik memurus*. An "other" category was included with instructions that the respondent should identify indigenous workers by title. It was felt that this approach would elicit some information about religious leaders, sorcerers, lead-pourers, bloodletters, etc., without detracting from the responses in the stated categories. However, because the initiative was left to the respondent, a significant under-reporting was expected in the "other" category.

Data were obtained on 31,802 villages, which were summarized according to the sixty-seven provinces and the eight statistical regions. A one-factor analysis of variance was conducted to verify the homogeneity of regional data. Similarity of the provincial data within each region was confirmed and, therefore, results are presented by statistical regions.

Because indigenous health practice in Turkey is illegal, our first concern was whether enough village leaders would agree to answer the questions to make the study meaningful and representative. Since responses were obtained from 90 percent of all villages, representing 88 percent of the population, the data are considered to be representative. The response rate by regions was consistently high.

Distribution of Rural Health Workers

The two categories of trained health workers were included in the survey to provide a check on reporting and so that this data could be compared with Ministry of Health records.

Significant net under-reporting was found in the rural health workers survey in both categories and in almost all statistical regions (Table 6–1). The 13 percent under-reporting of midwives could be because the activities of some midwives might be so limited that the village leader was not aware of their presence in his village. Another reasonable explanation for the discrepancy is that midwives may be reassigned frequently or may themselves migrate to

TABLE 6–1. COMPARISON OF NUMBER OF TRAINED MIDWIVES AND *Saglik Memurus* IN RURAL AREAS BY STATISTICAL REGIONS—DATA DERIVED FROM RURAL HEALTH WORKERS SURVEY AND MINISTRY OF HEALTH RECORDS, 1963

Statistical region	Trained midwives		*Saglik memurus*	
	Min. of health records	Health survey	Min. of health records	Health survey
Turkey in Europe	384	243	329	74
Black Sea coast	542	564	431	255
Marmara and Aegean Sea coasts	928	772	565	336
Mediterranean Sea coast	237	188	365	172
West Anatolia	343	342	332	204
Central Anatolia	712	613	832	307
Southeast Anatolia	84	84	143	73
East Anatolia	395	393	454	175
Total	3,625	3,199	3,451	1,596

the cities, and Ministry of Health records may not have been up to date in indicating their actual location at the time of the census. Since the Ministry records were found to be highly inaccurate for doctors, the latter is the more probable explanation.

The marked and widespread under-reporting of *saglik memurus*, however, is less readily explained. Village leaders reported the presence of only 46.2 percent of the *saglik memurus* that government records indicated should be in the villages. A question must be raised as to their effectiveness if the village leaders do not even report their presence. Again, a possible alternative explanation is that some may actually live in urban areas and commute to their assigned villages. Villagers, therefore, might not consider them resident workers. Whatever the explanation, these figures add to the evidence that the training, responsibility, and work relationships of *saglik memurus* must be clarified if they are to function effectively in villages.

The possibility of multiple counting of traditional health workers who serve more than one village is a potential limitation on the reliability of the survey findings. However, the under-reporting of trained health workers suggests that in this survey under-reporting will probably offset any such possible over-reporting. An over-reporting error is further minimized by the fact that 82 percent of all reported traditional health workers fall into two large groups— *ebe annes* and needlemen—who generally limit their practice to one village. Therefore, it is probable that net biases in the data are toward under-reporting.

The numbers in each of the traditional categories are summarized in Table 6–2, and the total comes to the impressive figure of 85,643.

These large numbers show the magnitude of the total health contribution of traditional health workers. Their presence cannot be ignored or brushed aside as irrelevant. As doctors assume greater responsibility in villages, they will find that their public relations will benefit if they control their prejudices and develop a positive relationship with this group. It will certainly be most difficult for doctors to adjust to dealing with those traditional health workers who are given the title of "doctor" and who actually examine, diagnose, and treat patients, using a mixture of traditional and modern medical methods.

A fundamental determinant which obviously influences the density of traditional health workers relative to trained workers is the degree of isolation of the rural area. No direct information about

TABLE 6–2. NUMBER OF TRADITIONAL HEALTH WORKERS BY STATISTICAL REGIONS, RURAL HEALTH WORKERS SURVEY, 1963

Statistical region	Types and no. of traditional health workers				
	Ebe anne	Needle-man	Circum-ciser	Bone-setter	Others[a]
Turkey in Europe	1,285	1,758	41	232	88
Black Sea coast	8,579	7,757	233	2,029	782
Marmara and Aegean Sea coasts	4,541	5,735	189	1,233	325
Mediterranean Sea coast	3,437	3,277	79	1,001	158
West Anatolia	3,142	3,207	152	1,194	440
Central Anatolia	8,629	5,839	271	2,654	485
Southeast Anatolia	1,926	584	30	1,091	34
East Anatolia	8,192	2,118	459	2,098	339
Total	39,731	30,275	1,454	11,532	2,651

[a] There were 2,405 tooth-pullers, 215 bloodletters, 22 umbilicus-setters, and 9 coccyx-pullers in the "others" group. Marked under-reporting was expected in this group.

the relative isolation of villages was available, but rates of literacy were. It is a safe generalization that the more isolated the area, the lower the literacy rate.

As areas become less isolated, trained health workers move in to replace traditional health workers. In Table 6–3 the statistical regions are ranked in order of literacy to show the correlation between the rate of literacy and the ratio of *ebe annes* to trained midwives. The ratio of *ebe annes* to trained midwives correlated inversely with the literacy rate and the relationship is statistically significant. The higher the literacy rate, the lower the ratio of *ebe annes* to trained midwives.

A marked difference was found in the relationships between the numbers of needlemen and of *ebe annes* and the literacy rate (Table 6–4). The distribution of needlemen correlates well with the literacy rate and the relationship is statistically significant. Where literacy rates are higher, more needlemen are to be found. The distribution of *ebe annes* shows almost no correlation with literacy, probably because the demand for obstetrical service remains relatively constant in a local population. There are not yet enough trained mid-

TABLE 6–3. COMPARISON OF EBE ANNES, TRAINED MIDWIVES, AND LITERACY RATES IN DIFFERENT REGIONS OF TURKEY, RURAL HEALTH WORKERS SURVEY, 1963

Statistical region	No. of midwives	No. of *ebe annes*	Ratio of *ebe anne* to TMW	Literacy rate in village	Ratio of *ebe anne* to TMW	Literacy
					Rank order	
Turkey in Europe	243	1,285	5.3	54	8	1
Marmara and Aegean Sea coasts	772	4,541	5.9	40	7	2
West Anatolia	342	3,142	9.2	35	6	3
Mediterranean Sea coast	188	3,437	18.3	30	3	4
Black Sea coast	564	8,579	15.2	26	4	5
Central Anatolia	613	8,629	14.1	25	5	6
East Anatolia	393	8,192	20.8	18	2	7
Southeast Anatolia	84	1,926	22.9	12	1	8
Total	3,199	39,731	12.4			

Rank order correlations: Ratio of *ebe annes* to trained midwives v. literacy $R = -.90$ (significant).

wives to have displaced them. On the other hand, the needleman provides a wide spectrum of services which in themselves increase local demand. His acceptance depends on his ability to provide a variety of treatments and supplies including injectables, ointments, oral medications, and various scientific devices which means that he must have access to urban centers to obtain supplies. It also takes a relatively affluent clientele to pay for these cash supplies. The needleman is a doctor substitute and precursor. The more contact a population has with urban centers, the more they will know about modern medicine, and, until doctors become available, these greater expectations will lead to greater demand for needlemen. Since both economic level and accessibility are correlated with literacy rate, the further close correlation with density of needlemen is readily explained. An additional reason for finding more needlemen in the less isolated areas is that the brighter and at least partially educated young men are usually chosen for training as medical corpsmen in the Army or for work in hospitals in cities. Therefore, fewer village youths from areas where literacy is low have the background training appropriate for such selection.

TABLE 6–4. DISTRIBUTION OF *Ebe Annes* AND NEEDLEMEN BY STATISTICAL REGIONS RANKED FOR COMPARISON WITH LITERACY RATE WITH RANK-ORDER CORRELATIONS, RURAL HEALTH WORKERS SURVEY, 1963

Statistical region	Literacy rate in villages (%)	No. of needle-men per village	No. of *ebe annes* per village	Rank order		
				Literacy	Needle-men	*Ebe anne*
Turkey in Europe	54	1.85	1.35	1	1	3
Marmara and Aegean Sea coasts	40	1.26	1.00	2	4	8
West Anatolia	35	1.21	1.18	3	5	6
Mediterranean Sea coast	30	1.48	1.56	4	2	1
Black Sea coast	26	1.34	1.48	5	3	2
Central Anatolia	25	0.74	1.10	6	6	7
East Anatolia	18	0.32	1.27	7	8	5
Southeast Anatolia	12	0.39	1.31	8	7	4
Average	29	0.95	1.24			

Rank order correlations: Literacy vs. Needlemen $R = .79$ (Significant)
Literacy vs. *Ebe Annes* $R = .05$ (Not Significant)
Needlemen vs. *Ebe Annes* $R = -.50$ (Not Significant)

Comparison of the distribution of bone-setters with literacy rates indicates that somewhat more bone-setters are found in remote areas where literacy rates are low and modern health services lacking. This relationship is not, however, sufficient to be statistically significant ($R = -.55$).

AVERAGE NUMBER OF TRADITIONAL HEALTH WORKERS IN A RURAL HEALTH CENTER AREA

From the total numbers of traditional workers found in the rural health workers survey, calculations have been made of the numbers that the staff of a rural health center in the Nationalized Health Program can expect to find in their area. It is assumed that a rural health center will serve about ten villages and a population of 7,000 —10,000. In this area there will probably be:

1. at least one *ebe anne* in each village;

2. approximately one needleman per village;
3. at least four bone-setters for the area;
4. one circumciser for the area;
5. one tooth-puller for the area;
6. possibly one mystic or religious healer for the area.

FACTORS INFLUENCING THE RELATIONSHIPS BETWEEN TRAINED AND TRADITIONAL HEALTH WORKERS

The trained health worker enters a village with the prestige and respect reserved for those who are educated and usually with the authority of official status. By contrast traditional health workers have long been accepted as part of the village social environment and often have considerable personal status. Many traditional healers practice on a part-time basis and, therefore, the arrival of a trained health worker is usually not so much an economic threat as a challenge to their social position and authority. Economically the official health workers are secure since they are subsidized by the government and therefore not dependent financially on the community. Usually, however, the new trained health worker is young, which is a distinct disadvantage in a society where age automatically commands respect and authority. Since the trained health worker is usually from an area with different customs, and often from a city, he will probably have personal as well as professional difficulties in adjusting to the village people and gaining their confidence.

The strong influence of social habit is based on generations of static traditional culture. Since many illnesses heal themselves anyway, it takes a dramatic cure to enable villagers to recognize qualitative differences in medical care. In times of illness, patients and their families feel an intrinsic insecurity and, therefore, they tend to seek medical help from a familiar person whose response can be readily anticipated. Oftentimes, the indigenous health worker's greatest success is in treating psychiatric and psychosomatic illnesses.

The *ebe anne* will probably continue to be progressively replaced as trained midwives are provided. But this will take many years. Serious consideration must be given to the possibility of using these women as recruiting agents in the National Family-Planning Program. A system of paying them for women they bring in for insertion of intrauterine contraceptive devices and other family-planning measures has been shown to work in countries such as Korea and Pakistan.

The needlemen probably depend on medical practice for a considerable part of their income. They readily adopt new medical methods that have gained popular acceptance. If they recognize a personal and professional advantage, they will probably be eager to take upgraded training so that they can be used in the health services. A promising proposal is that a joint training program be developed with the Army followed by an orientation course under the Ministry of Health. By using the required period of military service to train large numbers of rural health auxiliaries, a major manpower pool for the much-needed low-level rural auxiliary workers can be tapped.

The possibility of using other categories of traditional workers will be briefly summarized:

Circumcisers—The rather specialized combination of religious and health functions performed by these men are sufficiently limited so that they can serve a number of villages. In some areas they have already been replaced by *saglik memurus*. Because circumcisers travel a great deal and because of the religious overtones of circumcision, it may be difficult to regulate and upgrade their work.

Bone-setters—These highly specialized indigenous workers have no scientifically based knowledge. They rely primarily on manipulative skills and immobilization in treatment. Their greatest weakness is in diagnosis, especially for questionable fractures. Because prolonged healing is expected in fractures, there is ample time for varied and bizarre treatments to be applied before patients seek professional medical care. In obvious fractures, malunion or nonunion is frequent. However, a few bone-setters develop a wide reputation because of some dramatic successes. It will be difficult to upgrade the bone-setters or to utilize them effectively.

Tooth-pullers—This function may be performed by any of the traditional health workers. Acute toothache demands immediate care by anyone offering to help. As trained health workers become more available to villagers, these services will be provided more efficiently and these practitioners will disappear.

Religious teachers—The primary concern of these individuals is their religious function. No other group contributes as much, however, to dealing with psychiatric and psychosomatic illnesses. The introduction of trained health workers should be no threat to these practitioners. With the proper approach, their co-operation can be enlisted in improving the health care of the village.

Mystic healers, bloodletters, coccyx-pullers, umbilicus-setters—
This group of practitioners defies any clear classification because of
their varied sources of "power" and specialized techniques of treatment. They will probably continue to practice in the villages of
Turkey as their counterparts do in all countries. The relationship
of the trained health worker to these practitioners will necessarily
have to be on an invididual basis.

When an effort is made to incorporate traditional health workers
into organized health services, some form of training will be needed.
This may range from certificate courses to in-service training. Use
of these personnel will normally be on an interim basis until
more qualified individuals are available. Absorption into the rural
health services will have to be flexible and individualized with only
the most promising being selected. The best prospects for success
are with those categories which are already numerous and active
and who have the incentive of making sufficient income from health
work so that extra study and effort will be worth their while.

Trained health workers need to gain the respect of the villagers in
spite of the fact that they necessarily interrupt established social
patterns. Although change tends to be traumatic in any traditional
society, trained health workers should not appear unnecessarily
critical of the old ways. They should develop a positive approach
rather than deliberately undercutting the prestige of respected indigenous practitioners. Some of these respected traditional health
workers may be included in local health committees or given a voluntary function in rural health center programs. These possibilities
presuppose that the government will be less rigorous in enforcing
the present categorical legal prohibition of traditional health workers and will recognize their *de facto* existence during the necessary
transitional period.

In summary, the two categories of traditional workers who seem
most promising for continued use in the health services are the *ebe
annes* and the medical corpsmen who became needlemen. The *ebe
annes* may, for instance, be employed to recruit for the National
Family-Planning Program. They may also be given intensive simple
training to improve their handling of obstetrical cases. In a co-
operative program with the Army an effort can be made to use the
required military service for intensive training of medical auxiliaries.

7

ORGANIZATION AND ADMINISTRATION OF HEALTH SERVICES

The implementation of health manpower planning, especially within the short-range targets of the usual five-year plan, depends mainly on improved utilization of health personnel already available. Training programs to significantly augment supply require at least a fifteen-year planning period.

This study is concerned primarily with defining factors influencing the long-term supply-demand balance of health personnel. This chapter, however, describes the administrative framework of health services. Although official administrative patterns obviously determine the utilization of personnel employed in the public sector, there are many ways in which the private sector also is directly influenced. An understanding of the general administrative structure and functioning of health services is particularly relevant in Turkey because all projections depend primarily on government plans. Most significant is the potential impact of the new Plan for Nationalization of Health Services.

The Ministry of Health is responsible for improving the health conditions of the country, with activities divided in the traditional categories of public health and medical care services. The public health services are strictly the responsibility of the Ministry of Health with implementation delegated to municipal and local health authorities. There are 67 provincial directorates of health; local medical officers of health maintain 591 offices; municipal doctors maintain 230 offices; and there are 28 departments for malaria eradication.

Calculation of the relative responsibility of various agencies for medical care was based on their provision of hospital beds. Using this criterion, 52 percent of the medical care services are supported by the Ministry of Health and 27 percent by other ministries. The remainder is divided among philanthropic organizations (8 percent), Social Insurance (6 percent), municipal and local authorities (5 percent), proprietary hospitals (2 percent), business and industry (0.2 percent). The limited contribution at the municipal and local levels is due to poor organization and lack of funds. The Ministry of Health has the authority to supervise the administrative arrangements and health standards of all health institutions except those operated by the Ministry of Defense.

MATERIAL AND METHODS

A list of all health institutions, except those operated by the Ministry of Defense, was obtained from the Ministry of Health. Questionnaires were sent to each institution, supplemented by personal interviews when indicated. Since information could be secured directly from the Ministry of Health about its own institutions and those operated by municipal and local authorities, they did not receive questionnaires. Replies were received on 367 of the 436 questionnaires which were sent out, for a response rate of 79.5 percent. Another source of information was a book entitled *Health Activities in the Republican Era*, written by Dr. Feridun Frik in 1964. This provided a cross-check list and also gave information about health institutions operated by the Ministry of Defense. The data represent the situation in May, 1964. A separate booklet listing the number and types of health institutions in Turkey was compiled from this health manpower study for immediate use by Ministry officials and other interested persons.

HEALTH INSTITUTIONS

Health Institutions which Belong to the Ministry of Health, Municipalities, and Local Authorities.

The administrative organization of the Ministry of Health is divided into two parts—central and provincial. The Ministry of Health is ultimately responsible for all health services. The Undersecretary is the chief executive officer and handles routine administration. Assistants to the undersecretary are in charge of various directorates such as tuberculosis control, family planning, and personnel.

Each province has a Director of Health appointed by the Ministry of Health. He is the highest health official in the province but is officially under the administrative control of the governor. Each province is divided into *kazas* or districts with a *kaymakam* as the highest administrative officer. In every *kaza* there is a medical officer of health who acts as health advisor to the *kaymakam*. In cities medical officers work directly under the Provincial Director of Health but in the *kazas* they are under the administrative control of the *kaymakam*. The Ministry of Health appoints municipality doctors but they are paid by the municipal authorities.

The medical care services performed by the Ministry of Health and municipal and local authorities are shown in Table 7–1. These include 717 hospitals and health centers with wards which have a total of 42,508 beds. The average bed capacity was 146 for hospitals and 13 for health centers.

In addition, most routine preventive services and a certain amount of ambulatory medical care are provided in institutions

TABLE 7–1. TYPES, NUMBER, AND BED CAPACITY OF HEALTH INSTITUTIONS OF THE MINISTRY OF HEALTH, MUNICIPALITIES, AND LOCAL AUTHORITIES,[a] 1964

Types of health institutions	Total number	Total bed capacity	Av. bed capacity
General hospitals	127	17,412	138
Specialty hospitals:			
Trachoma	7	165	24
Maternity and children's	33	4,285	129
Chest diseases	68	8,595	126
Leprosy	1	265	265
Mental	3	4,550	1,516
Cancer	1	75	75
Bone diseases	4	1,085	271
Venereal diseases	4	305	81
Rabies	4	105	26
Health centers (with bed)	295	3,943	13
Dispensaries (with bed) and			
Examination and treatment centers	158	866	6
Day nursery and orphanage	1	100	100
Home for the disabled and elderly	11	757	69
Total	717	42,508	59

[a] Of the total of 42,508 hospital beds, 38,838 beds belong to the Ministry of Health and 3,620 to municipalities and local authorities.

which do not have beds. These 1,114 institutions usually provide specialized services (Table 7–2).

TABLE 7–2. PUBLIC HEALTH INSTITUTIONS WITHOUT BEDS BELONGING TO THE
MINISTRY OF HEALTH, MUNICIPALITIES, AND LOCAL AUTHORITIES, 1964

Types of health institutions	Total no.
Health centers	8
Mother and child health centers (with branches)	88
Dispensaries	156
Health units (nationalization area)	18
Trachoma rural centers	202
Rabies vaccination stations	241
Mother and child health stations	360
Quarantine stations	3
Rehabilitation centers	8
Blood transfusion centers	19
Health museums	8
Day nurseries	3
Total	1,114

Health Institutions which Belong to Other Ministries, State Economic Enterprises, and Medical Schools

Approximately half of the medical care facilities owned and operated by the government are not directly under the Ministry of Health. Several ministries have their own medical care facilities for employees or special groups such as the armed forces. The state economic enterprises and medical schools have major responsibilities and considerable independence. The hospitals are almost twice the size of Ministry of Health hospitals, averaging 242 beds (Table 7–3).

Health Institutions which Belong to Social Insurance

Social insurance institutions provide health services for insured workers and their dependents. The facilities are primarily concentrated in industrialized urban areas (Table 7–4).

Places of employment have been required by law to provide health services since 1930. These requirements had been fairly well fulfilled by the state economic enterprises and by large private firms prior to 1946 when social insurance started. Since that time, social insurance has established outpatient departments and hospitals in many parts of the country, thus relieving industry of the

TABLE 7–3. NUMBER AND BED CAPACITY OF HEALTH INSTITUTIONS OPERATED
BY MINISTRIES OTHER THAN MINISTRY OF HEALTH IN TURKEY, 1964

Types of health institutions	Total no.	Total bed capacity	Av. bed capacity
General hospitals	67	14,035	204
Specialty hospitals:			
Chest Diseases	6	1,139	190
Teaching hospitals:			
(belonging to med. schools)	4	3,510	488
Health center (without bed)	1	—	—
Dispensaries (with bed)	11	153	14
Dispensaries (without bed)	2	—	—
Infirmaries (with bed)	51	984	19
Infirmaries (without bed)	4	—	—
Health unit (with bed)	1	25	25
Health unit (without bed)	10	—	—
Dental treatment center	1	—	—
Rehabilitation center	1	—	—
Center for the protection of workers' health	1	—	—
Day nurseries and orphanages	7	525	75
Total	167	20,371	130

TABLE 7–4. TYPES, TOTAL NUMBER, AND BED CAPACITY OF THE HEALTH
INSTITUTIONS OPERATED BY SOCIAL INSURANCE IN TURKEY, 1964

Types of health institutions	Total no.	Total bed capacity	Av. bed capacity
General hospital	27	3,489	129
Specialty hospital:			
Chest diseases	1	510	510
Maternity	2	135	68
Dispensary:			
With bed	2	42	21
Without Bed	22	—	—
Health station	27	—	—
Dental treatment center	1	—	—
Total	82	4,176	51

responsibility. By 1964, insurance benefits covered only 680,000
workers. In 1965 a new comprehensive Social Insurance Law replaced the old programs which will expand coverage to include
some two and a half million dependents as well as workers.

Proprietary Health Institutions

In urban areas there are a few small private hospitals and clinics which are operated primarily for profit. They all have permanent auxiliary staff, but many do not have full-time doctors. Any private practitioner may treat his own patients in these institutions. The patient pays a fee directly to his private doctor and the hospital costs to the private hospital (Table 7–5).

TABLE 7–5. PROPRIETARY HEALTH INSTITUTIONS IN TURKEY, 1964

Types of health institutions	No. of health institutions	Bed capacity	Av. bed capacity
General hospitals or clinics	38	835	22
Specialty hospitals:			
Maternity	7	134	19
Chest diseases	8	580	73
Mental	1	24	24
Total	54	1,573	29

Health Institutions Operated by Business and Industry

There are still some private firms providing health services for their own personnel. Most of these companies employ private doctors on a contract basis and when an employee requires hospitalization his firm pays for the hospital services. The only health institutions still run by industries are a hospital with 151 beds, another with 10 beds, an infirmary with 13 beds, and a dispensary with 20 beds.

Health Institutions which Belong to Philanthropic Organizations

Certain health establishments are nonprofit institutions operated by voluntary and philanthropic organizations. Those for Turkish minority groups are mainly in Istanbul, while those operated by foreign agencies tend to be somewhat more dispersed but, again, they are mainly urban (Table 7–6).

PLANS FOR REORGANIZATION OF HEALTH SERVICES

Nationalization of Health Services

General dissatisfaction with the rate of health improvement led to recognition of the need for a bold approach to the reorganization

TABLE 7–6. TYPES, TOTAL NUMBER, AND BED CAPACITY OF HEALTH INSTITUTIONS
OPERATED BY PHILANTHROPIC ORGANIZATIONS IN TURKEY IN 1964

Types of health institutions	Total no.	Total bed capacity	Av. bed capacity
General hospitals	16	1,825	114
Specialty hospitals:			
Chest diseases	2	314	157
Maternity	1	10	10
Mental	1	150	150
Dispensaries (without bed)	61	—	—
Day nurseries and orphanages	30	2,601	86
Home for the disabled and elderly	5	784	156
Rehabilitation centers	4	—	—
Outpatient centers	9	—	—
Total	129	5,684	84[a]

[a] Dispensaries without beds are not included in the average.

of health services. In January, 1961, a law was passed setting up a nationalized health service that, within a fifteen-year period, was to cover the entire country with a complete network of preventive and curative services. Because of the gross geographic maldistribution of services, much of the initial effort was devoted to equalization of health services for the neglected 70 percent of the population who live in rural areas.

The law provides for regionalization of provincial health services. Each region of the country has three to six provinces and will have a minimum of one hospital with 400 to 500 beds and one public health laboratory. The Director of Health for each province has a deputy director and heads of special services (malaria, trachoma, tuberculosis, etc.). Each province is divided into health areas with about 100,000 inhabitants which will be served by a hospital with approximately 100 beds.

Major attention in the nationalized health plan is concentrated on providing both curative and preventive services through a system of rural health centers. Each center is to serve 7,000 to 10,000 people and have three to five satellite health stations, each serving a population of about 2,000 people. The health center is staffed by a doctor (general practitioner), a nurse, a *saglik memuru*, a clerk (medical secretary), a driver, and a janitor. The satellite stations are each staffed by a rural midwife and are under the regular supervision and support of the health center staff. To provide a link between health areas and the provincial health directorate a senior physician is designated as co-ordinator. He is usually the medical director of the hospital in the health area.

In 1963, the new nationalized health services was started on a pilot basis in one eastern province (Mus), and was extended to five more provinces in 1964. The anticipated sequence for implementing the nationalized health plan by provinces is shown in Table 7–7 but present indications are that the rate of expansion will have to be delayed.

TABLE 7–7. PHASED PROGRAM FOR THE NATIONALIZED HEALTH SERVICES OF TURKEY, INDICATING THE YEAR WHEN EACH PROVINCE WILL BE INCLUDED

Year	Provinces
1963	Mus
1964	Hakkari, Bitlis, Van, Agri, Kars
1965	Erzurum, Erzincan, Diyarbakir, Siirt, Mardin, Urfa
1966	Tunceli, Bingol, Elazig, Adiyaman, Malatya, Artvin, Gumushane
1967	Rize, Trabzon, Giresun, Maras
1968	Kayseri, Sivas, Tokat, Amasya
1969	Corum, Yozgat, Kireshir, Nevsehir, Nigde
1970	Ordu, Samsun, Sinop, Gasiantep, Hatay
1971	Adana, Icel, Konya
1972	Kastamonu, Bolu, Cankiri, Ankara
1973	Eskisehir, Afyon, Bilecik, Kutahya, Usak, Isparta, Burdur
1974	Antalya, Mugla, Kocaeli, Sakarya, Zonguldak
1975	Denizli, Aydin, Izmir, Manisa
1976	Bursa, Balikesir, Canakkale
1977	Istanbul, Tekirdag, Edirne, Kirklareli

As the plan is implemented all the health institutions in the public sector, except the Ministry of Defense, will be taken over by the unified administration. Private practitioners and private health institutions will be left free to generate their own support and develop as they can.

According to the regulations of the nationalized health services, patients pay nothing for routine health services but, except in an emergency, they are charged for special drugs. When doctors are called outside of working hours, and especially for home calls, they can charge fees according to scales set by the Ministry of Health and this money must be paid to the government Treasury. Patients sent to the hospital through the health unit pay nothing, but patients who go to the hospital on their own are charged. Spectacles, dentures, and appliances are not provided. It is expected that some kind of social insurance will gradually develop to provide a major part of the finances for the nationalized health plan. Meanwhile all expenses are being paid from the government budget.

To attract health personnel, a three-year contract was offered at three to four times the regular government salary scale. Base pay in liras ranges from 675 TL ($75) per month, with increments at three-year intervals to a thirty-year scale of 2700 TL ($300). In addition, allowances are provided for private practice, hardship posts, and mobile work which range from 1000 ($111) to 2000 TL ($222). Specialists get an additional 700 TL ($77). Doctors must work full time and are not allowed private practice. *Saglik memurus*, nurses, and other paramedical staff received similar relative increases in pay. The base pay ranges from 405 TL ($45) to 2,020 TL ($225) with supplements ranging from 200 TL ($22) to 2000 TL ($222).

Integrated Health Services

When the plan for nationalization of health services was started in 1963, a special plan was formulated to provide less intensive health services for those areas where the benefits of the new nationalization plan would not extend for many years. It seemed hardly appropriate to leave rural areas in most of Turkey essentially neglected while the total program gradually expanded. This plan was designed to be eventually incorporated into the expanding nationalization plan so that ultimately all of Turkey will have the same rural health organization.

Priority in starting the integrated health services is given to areas where malaria eradication is reaching the surveillance phase. Malaria workers can, therefore, be absorbed into general public health activities. There is a central administrative office in the provincial health directorate to control all existing services and to make more efficient use of any additional manpower which may be added from time to time.

The plan provides that each province be divided into health areas serving 37,500 persons. Each such area is to be served by one general practitioner, one health technician, one midwife, and one malaria surveillance chief. To function within the health areas are health units serving 7,500 persons. Each unit will be staffed by one malaria surveillance agent, one *saglik memuru*, and one midwife. The health units are to be further divided into health stations with 2,500 people. One rural midwife is to serve each station. The major emphasis is obviously on services provided by auxiliaries.

All types of health personnel within each department are required to visit the villages according to a specified schedule. The focus is primarily on preventive services such as improvement of environmental sanitation, vaccination, health education, and maternal and child health care.

An integral part of the system is that doctors working in government hospitals and health institutions throughout the province will be required to visit the health units nearest them to provide curative health services in outpatient clinics. These visits are to follow a schedule set up by the provincial health director. The village people are expected to provide buildings for the health units and health stations. Equipment and motor vehicles are supplied by UNICEF.

Quality of Care Provided under Nationalized Health Service

A pilot project is useful only if it is evaluated. Since the nationalization of health services started in pilot form in the province of Mus in 1963, a Turkish member of the health manpower team conducted an evaluation of the project in June, 1964, ten months after the project started. Quality judgments were largely subjective. Considerable data were, however, gathered from routine records which permit some objective comparisons with pre-existing services.

For the purposes of this study, if it could be demonstrated that the health services in Mus had been improved in a worthwhile manner, it would strengthen greatly the rationale of basing further planning on the nationalization plan. For manpower projections, the standardized pattern of staffing health centers would greatly simplify the process of projecting demand for health personnel. Manpower demand curves then would merely require simple arithmetic calculations based on personnel/population ratios and known demographic trends.

The first finding was a quantitative increase in the number of health personnel (Table 7–8). The most dramatic increase was in the number of auxiliary health personnel which increased from 35 to 123. There were 18 health units and 42 subunits in the province.

TABLE 7–8. POPULATION PER DIFFERENT TYPES OF HEALTH PERSONNEL BEFORE AND AFTER NATIONALIZATION OF HEALTH SERVICES IN THE PROVINCE OF MUS, 1964 EVALUATION

Type of health personnel	Before nationalization (1962)[a]		After nationalization (1963)[b]	
	No. of health personnel	Pop. per health personnel	No. of health personnel	Pop. per health personnel
Specialists	2	90,066	12	15,531
General practitioners	8	22,516	23	8,103
Asst. health personnel	35	5,147	123	1,515
Dentists	1	180,132	2	93,189
Pharmacists	1	180,132	1	186,379
Total	47	3,832	161	1,158

[a] Estimated population of the province of Mus in 1962 was 180,132.
[b] Estimated population of the province of Mus in 1963 was 186,379.

More important than increased manpower were the expanded medical services. One indication was the markedly increased utilization. During 1962, total outpatients treated in institutions or at home was 13,000. In 1963 the first year of operation of the full nationalization plan, this number went up to 122,601 (Figure 7–1). Of this number, 105,883 were seen in health units and of these, 6,782 patients were referred to hospitals for examination by specialists. In addition, there were 16,718 patients who went directly to the hospitals for care. The most important consideration is that 81 percent of the patients who required care were treated in health units without referral to hospitals.

Hospital care also increased markedly as a result of the nationalized health program. The 3,271 patients admitted for inpatient hospitalization in 1963 were more than twice the total inpatients treated in 1962 (Figure 7–1). There was no increase in the number of beds, but the bed occupancy rate was 50 percent in 1962 as compared to 96.5 percent in 1963. During the same year the number of surgical operations performed in Mus hospitals went up from 187 to 440.

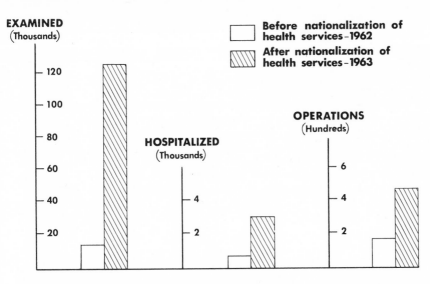

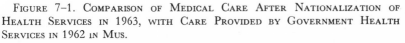

Figure 7–1. Comparison of Medical Care After Nationalization of Health Services in 1963, with Care Provided by Government Health Services in 1962 in Mus.

Most of the preventive services are administratively part of the responsibility of health units. An estimated 56 percent of the total annual health expenditure of all health units in the province was devoted to preventive activities. Another evidence of the amount of preventive work is the large number of visits to peripheral villages by health personnel. In an average month 1,373 villages were visited by 101 health workers. If no two health personnel visited the same village, this means that each of them traveled to about 14 different villages per month. It is probable that there was considerable overlap and, if so, the number of villages visited per person would be even more impressive.

One of the most important services provided by hospital specialists was that they all visited health units two days a week in order to provide general practitioners with professional support. The lists of diseases cared for in the health centers indicates concentration on the primary health problems of the area. The diseases most frequently seen were infant diarrhea, malnutrition, pneumonia, other communicable diseases, and accidents.

Maternal and child health services were provided mainly by rural midwives. The fifty-two midwives working in the area made

82,400 house visits; they found 8,915 pregnancy cases and conducted 2,578 deliveries. If the birthrate in this part of Turkey is 50 per 1,000 population, 30 percent of the deliveries of the area were conducted by midwives. For the first year of the program this is a remarkable achievement.

The *saglik memurus* employed in the health units bore most of the responsibility for communicable disease control under the direction of health unit doctors and the provincial health director. Particular emphasis was placed on the vaccination program. In 1962 before nationalization the following vaccinations were administered: typhoid—31,210, whooping cough—6,500, and diphtheria—6,635. In the year after nationalization, the following vaccinations were administered: poliomyelitis—77,425, typhoid—100,782, diphtheria—37,303, whooping cough—17,883, tetanus—5,461, smallpox—4,726, and BCG—685. *Saglik memurus* made 7,628 visits to houses and 2,591 to schools and public places to improve sanitary conditions; in addition, approximately 2,000 latrines were inspected.

Great effort went into health education with 11,844 persons being included in group education and 138,278 being contacted individually. All members of the health unit staff were included in these educational activities.

The expansion of specific disease contol activities is indicated by the following figures. Starting in August, 1963, the 140 persons with syphilis and 531 persons with leprosy, known from previous surveys, were registered and periodic examination and treatment initiated. Another 25 individuals with leprosy who were diagnosed during a survey of the area were registered and put under control. An eye specialist conducted village surveys and diagnosed 4,682 trachoma cases, of which 1,849 were placed on regular treatment. An additional 3,842 conjunctivitis cases were diagnosed and treated.

The health units will be responsible for the "passive surveillance" phase of the malaria eradication program. Malaria eradication in Mus is now in the "attack phase" with 99.4 percent of houses sprayed with DDT. Blood examinations were done on 2,294 persons and 66 malaria cases were found. Tuberculosis control in the area has been accelerated. A special mobile screening unit and BCG team completed Mantoux tuberculin testing of 98 percent of the population. They administered BCG vaccinations to 73,788 persons within a two-month perod in the fall of 1963. Chest microfilms of 7,588 persons with suspicious findings identified 214 new cases of tuberculosis who were placed under treatment in the Tuberculosis Control Dispensary. Also, chest x-rays of 17,520 persons were made by the central provincial Tuberculosis Control Dispensary.

Cost of Nationalized Health Services

The per capita cost of the nationalized health services is low. In 1963, the annual per capita health expenditure in Mus was 32 TL ($3.55). Compared with health expenditures in other Turkish agencies and foreign countries, this is a modest figure. For example, the annual health expenditure per capita is $15 in Israel, $44.44 in Sweden, and even in Ceylon the per capita expenditure is $3.22. The annual health expenditure per insured worker of the Turkish Workers' Insurance Institutions is 151 TL ($16.77) (see Figure 7–2).

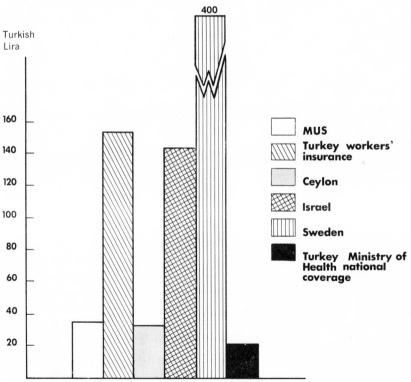

Figure 7–2. Health Expenditures Per Capita in Selected Countries, as Compared with Nationalized Health Services in Mus and Other Turkish Health Services.

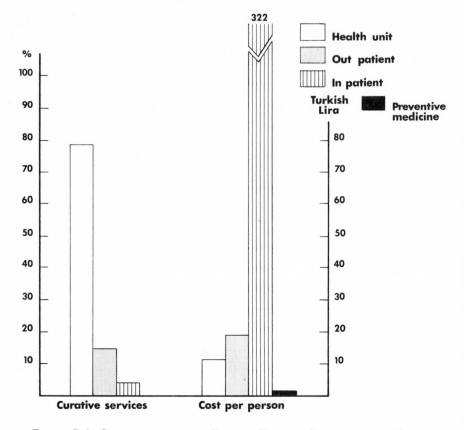

FIGURE 7–3. COMPARISON OF THE COST OF VARIOUS COMPONENTS OF HEALTH
SERVICES IN MUS, 1963.

A comparison of curative services performed in health centers
and hospitals in Mus in 1963 shows that the health units handled
80 percent of the patient load (Figure 7–3).

The annual health expenditure for all health units in the province was 2,889,000 TL ($321,000). Of this, the expenditure on
curative health services was 1,275,000 TL ($141,666). The cost of
treating one patient was 12 TL. The annual expenditure on hospital services was 1,667,000 TL ($185,222). The cost of outpatient
health services per patient was 16 TL ($1.77), and the cost of in-
patient health services per patient was 322 TL ($35.78) (see Figure
7–3). The per person expenditure on preventive medicine services
in directorates and health units was 1.1 TL (12¢).

According to calculations based on the Mus experience, the cost of nationalization of health services for the whole country would be 6 percent of the national budget. This slight increase in cost above the present proportion should be considered in the perspective of the remarkable increase in clinical care (up from 13,000 patient visits to 122,601 in one year), and the considerable improvement of preventive and community health services. The cost is small relative to the great benefit.

Recommendations for Changes in Nationalized Health Services

The following recommendations for modification of the nationalized services were made as a result of this evaluation of the Mus pilot project:

(a) Health services require better co-ordination with other official departments, especially community development services.

(b) Even though a considerable effort has been made in public health education, all personnel should be even more involved and should be given training in the use of educational equipment.

(c) Health personnel living in villages or small towns require special arrangements for food and improved amenities for decent living. These personal needs must be met to maintain recruitment.

(d) More equitable practices should be established for the assignment and rotation of health personnel so that after a period of service of about three years in a remote area an individual could be reassigned to a place of his choice. These policies should be followed faithfully and consistently.

(e) The construction of health units should be adapted to the climatic conditions of the area rather than being rigidly standardized as at present.

(f) Health units should be located in villages and towns which are convenient for the most people, with special attention to transportation routes.

(g) The central organization of the Ministry of Health should be reorganized with even greater provision of flexible arrangements and experimental approaches for meeting the special needs of the provinces where the health services are being nationalized.

(h) Health units and health subunits should be provided with telephones and running water.

(i) Health unit doctors should be given special training, with appropriate field experience, to prepare them for both curative and preventive responsibilities at appropriate periods in medical school, after graduation, and in-service.

(j) Because of the limited resources of the Ministry of Health, more importance should be attached to effective implementation and improvement of the quality of health services already established rather than moving ahead with nationwide expansion too rapidly and methods should be developed of getting greater community involvement in financing local health services.

In summary, the most important achievement of the nationalized services in Mus Province was in reaching a large proportion of the population with the limited facilities of the health units. Ninety-seven percent of patients were treated in the outpatient departments of health units and hospitals or at home. The plan also improved utilization of health personnel. Health services were taken out to the villages with regular visits by all categories of personnel. It was the subjective impression of our team that villagers were satisfied with the services. Local newspapers also expressed satisfaction over the fact that patients now get service from doctors instead of indigenous healers. The Mus experience demonstrated that under appropriate conditions doctors and other health personnel could live and work successfully in villages.

THE MINISTRY OF HEALTH BUDGET

Throughout this research project particular attention has been paid to economic feasibility. For the first time in Turkey, studies were done to gather and analyze date on the costs of such basic activities as medical education, hospital services, and private practice. Much effort went into gathering original data. Methodological innovations in analysis were necessary. It is recognized that many of the final calculations are not accurate and are only first approximations which will require further refinement. Even as first approximations, however, they provide a more valid basis for judgments on manpower planning.

While our study was being done the planning unit of the Ministry of Health also undertook to analyze and project health service costs in a document published in 1964 by the Ankara School of Public Health.[1] This report used basic information available in official records. Interpretations were made by an expert group of physicians and economists from the Ministry of Health, the State Planning Organization, and the Ankara School of Public Health. Because their estimates still represent a synthesis of the best expert opinion available, they have been accepted as a preliminary basis for our calculations.

The over-all distribution of the Ministry's financial allocations in 1964 is shown in Table 7–9. Hospital expenditures were 47.3 percent of total expenditures. Only 11.7 percent was actually spent on health centers in comparison with 16.1 percent allocated. An impressive 17.2 percent was spent for contagious diseases, to which should be added 4.1 percent for tuberculosis control.

TABLE 7–9. THE BUDGET[a] OF THE MINISTRY OF HEALTH AND SOCIAL WELFARE (1964)
(1,000 TL)

Projects	Personnel costs (budgeted)	Total expenses		% distribution of total allocations	
		Budgeted	Actually expended	Budgeted	Actually expended
Health centers	26,570	141,518	79,722	16.1	11.7
Hospitals	252,809	431,579	322,731	48.8	47.3
TB	21,844	38,687	27,797	4.4	4.1
Public health labs	4,593	10,988	10,082	1.2	1.5
Maintenance	1,889	7,995	7,610	0.9	1.1
Health schools	21,381	65,115	54,603	7.4	8.0
Health ed. and med. statistics	153	400	400	0.05	0.06
Social services	8,637	24,529	17,419	2.8	2.6
MCH	10,600	13,740	13,740	1.6	2.0
Contagious diseases	96,361	118,373	118,774	13.4	17.2
Central organization	19,102	29,994	28,746	3.4	4.2
Total	442,095	883,918	681,626	—	—

[a] Fisek and Koksoy, Planning Unit of the Ministry of Health (Ankara School of Public Health, 1964).

Increases in the budget of the Ministry of Health and Social Welfare were projected up to 1977 by the planning unit of the Ministry (Table 7–10). Some impressive shifts were made, particularly the increase to 74 percent allocated to personnel in comparison with 50 percent in 1964. This figure indicates dramatically the tremendous importance attached to manpower planning.

TABLE 7–10. THE BUDGET OF THE MINISTRY OF HEALTH AND SOCIAL WELFARE (1977)
(1,000 TL)

Projects	Personnel costs (budgeted)	Total expenses Budgeted	% distribution of total allocations Budgeted
Health centers	537,380	673,656	33.7
Hospitals	660,974	876,881	43.9
TB	53,219	92,460	4.6
Public health labs	19,806	29,256	1.5
Maintenance	30,543	52,186	2.6
Health schools	34,228	60,449	3.0
Health ed. and med. statistics	1,390	2,667	0.1
Social services	15,628	29,684	1.5
MCH	15,081	22,085	1.1
Contagious diseases	75,497	99,794	5.0
Central organization	40,700	59,025	3.0
Total	1,484,446	1,998,143	—

Since the medical schools are under the Ministry of Education, they have not been included in the above calculations. Because our calculations of costs of medical education (Chapter 3, pp. 115–21) were preliminary and because there are still many uncertainties in projecting future expansion, we have not attempted to project costs of medical education. However, it is clear from the sharp increase in the total costs of medical education in the past ten years that it will become even more expensive.

Further specific calculations permit some extrapolation of medical care costs beyond the Ministry of Health budgets in Tables 7–9 and 7–10. Calculations from our data on hospital in-patients are as follows: in the detailed cost studies of ten selected hospitals, our calculations were that the average cost per hospital bed per day was 34 TL (Chapter 9). In 1964 there were 74,506 hospital beds in Turkey. This gives a total cost for all hospital beds of 2.5 million Turkish lira per day or over 900 million TL per year as compared with 471 million TL budgeted for all public beds and 322 million TL for Ministry of Health beds.

SUMMARY

The administrative framework of the government-supported health services of Turkey suffers from fragmentation. Various ministries and official agencies have their own systems of medical care. These are frequently competitive or conflicting. For instance, the initial successes of the nationalized health services in recruiting staff were because they paid about four times the regular government scale and really required full-time work. On the basis of this precedent other government agencies increased their salary scales. The nationalized health services then encountered the usual recruitment problems. Uniform policies should cover all government agencies with built-in provisions for appropriate local corrective mechanisms such as giving a liberal rural allowance.

Imaginative administrative reform can make major improvements in manpower utilization and distribution.

REFERENCE

1. Dr. Nusret H. Fisek and Col. Riza Koksoy, *Expenditures Necessary for the Nationalization of Health Services and the Finance of the Project*, Planning Unit of the Ministry of Health, Publication No. 14 (Ankara School of Public Health, 1964).

8

PROJECTED CHANGES IN SUPPLY OF HEALTH MANPOWER

The most important long-range objective of manpower planning is to plan the extent and nature of changes in the educational system. This requires careful projection of future supply and demand.

Skilled manpower can be obtained from the following sources:

1. Some of the necessary skills may be already available in the present stock of manpower if distribution could be improved, but the location as well as the magnitude of the gap between supply and demand must be clearly defined.

2. In some countries a temporary expedient is to import skilled manpower from abroad but this seems neither practical nor desirable in Turkey's present stage of advancement.

3. To fill short-term needs, it may be possible to substitute available types of personnel for those categories with the greatest shortages. A portion of the total manpower gap may be met by retraining and upgrading persons now qualified for less skilled occupations. In-service training can also improve the effectiveness of persons now underqualified for jobs they are already doing.

4. The greatest hidden resource in manpower planning is to improve utilization and productivity, especially by improving the balance between professionals and auxiliaries. The basic dictum is to limit the use of professionals to those tasks which only professionals can do and to use auxiliaries for all routine activities.

5. Ultimately, developing skilled manpower must be the responsibility of the formal educational system.

In projecting manpower supply the first step is to determine the balance between persons entering the manpower pool and those leaving it through retirement, death, emigration, or transferral to other activities. Increments occur only as there is a difference between inflow and outflow. The inflow is conditioned by several constraints such as the available educational pool, number of applicants, and the educational system itself.

HEALTH CATEGORIES FOR WHICH PROJECTIONS WERE NOT DONE

Detailed projections have been done for only four categories of health personnel—doctors, nurses, trained nurses' aides, and rural midwives. The indications are that these are the four in which prospective shortages are severe enough to require immediate planning and adjustment of the educational output.

Special categories such as dentists and pharmacists have not been included for several reasons: the supply-demand balance does not seem severely askew and spontaneous adjustments of educational productivity will probably meet demand as it expands; more than three-fourths of these professionals are employed in the private sector and are, therefore, less influenced by government planning; they are largely urban in distribution; and so far they have been included in planning for the Nationalized Health Services in only a minor way.

An obvious need which is inadequately documented is to develop auxiliary training programs for dental assistants and pharmacist assistants. The improvement of basic services in dentistry and pharmacy is greatly needed in public sector institutions. These functions should then become part of the tremendous expansion required in the above categories of health personnel.

Detailed projections on another major category of middle-level health personnel—*saglik memurus*—were not done because: this group seems to be relatively well supplied at the moment by the present output from educational institutions; there is no problem in attracting students for this training program so that if a shortage does develop, rapid expansion should be possible; even though the nationalization plan and the interim Integrated Plan of Health Services are to a large extent built on this category of health personnel, there is no indication that there will be difficulty filling the new positions; finally, the *saglik memuru* has never been carefully conceptualized in terms of functions to be carried out or role definition vis à vis other health personnel. He serves as a multipurpose worker, often in jobs for which he has not been trained. Until there is a clear definition of the role of the *saglik memuru*, it is difficult to project his position in future health services.

As indicated in the chapter on projections in demand, however, the supply of rural midwives will have to sharply increase to meet the requirements of the new nationalized health plans and the national family-planning program. The training of rural midwives has recently been shifted to the health schools. A massive expansion of this program will be necessary. A brief analysis of the rural midwife supply prospects, therefore, is included.

The greatest unrecognized deficiency in the health manpower requirements of Turkey is the almost complete lack of personnel specifically prepared to handle problems of environmental sanitation. The *saglik memuru* comes nearest to filling this role but his training is not sufficiently focused. He is also called on to fill such a diverse range of activities that he cannot give sanitation the concentrated attention it deserves. We are not implying that Turkey should necessarily develop the pattern of sanitary engineers and sanitarians existing in other countries. Turkey should, however, make its own approach to filling this major manpower deficiency.

Finally, there is a category of health worker who is usually ignored in official planning, even though they are the most numerous in Turkey. "Needlemen" now provide the bulk of medical care to rural people, among whom they are accepted as doctors. Their role needs attention.

PROJECTION OF DOCTOR SUPPLY

Methods of Calculation

Projections of physician supply were done for all doctors without special regard to the high rate of specialization. Shortages of general practitioners which are particularly great will not be specifically estimated. The basis of the calculations has been to develop standard increments to the present manpower pool on the basis of minimum and maximum assumptions and thus to arrive at figures expected in 1967, 1972, and 1977.

The basic input comes from total expected graduates of present medical schools. Some changes have occurred in recent years with Istanbul reducing the size of its classes and the other three schools gradually increasing their output. By averaging the five years before 1964, the following figures were obtained: Istanbul, 236 graduates per year; Ankara, 140 graduates per year; and Ege University (based on a three-year calculation), 66 graduates per year. Hacettepe was arbitrarily credited with 75 graduates per year. The total is 515 graduates per year. The number of graduates increased steadily after the 1920's but there has been a leveling off since the mid-1950's as the new schools have approximately compensated for the decrease in class size at Istanbul (Table 8–1). Since it seems reasonable for schools such as Izmir to increase admissions, a round-off figure of 540 graduates per year was used for these projections.

The first Five-Year Plan includes five new medical schools to be opened, mainly in smaller cities in the east. The most optimistic hopes are that two of these new schools may be turning out graduates between 1972 and 1977.

The attrition rate was calculated from estimates of deaths, retirements, and losses to other countries. Table 8–1 shows deaths of Turkish doctors by year of graduation and the numbers expected to be living in 1964.

TABLE 8–1. INCREMENTS TO TURKISH DOCTOR SUPPLY BY TEN-YEAR COHORTS BASED ON YEAR OF GRADUATION SINCE 1923[a]

Year of graduation	Average no. drs. graduated annually	Average no. dead from each annual cohort	Residual in annual cohort	Total number living
1923–9	78	28	50	350
1930–9	141	21	120	1,200
1940–9	400	14	386	3,860
1950–9	491	7	484	4,840
1960–3	455	0	455	1,820
Total				12,070

[a] The 188 graduates of non-Turkish medical schools are not included.

The principal increase of Turkish doctors occurred after 1940 when the average number of annual graduates abruptly jumped to 400. Estimating forty years of active professional life for a doctor, this means that up to 1980 attrition rates due to death would apply mainly to the relatively small pool of pre-1940 doctors. It seems reasonable, then, to estimate only slight increases in attrition rates for the interval up to 1977 included in our projections.

In 1964, Ministry of Health records as checked by our survey show that the following losses occurred: eighteen doctors died and twenty-one retired. To allow for slightly increasing attrition rates, we have used the approximation of fifty doctors per year dying and retiring. Projection with this figure becomes increasingly hazardous more than ten years from now, but so do all our other projections.

The second major source of doctor loss is from migration to foreign countries (Table 8–2). The final column in this table shows the total number of active doctors estimated to be residing in Turkey. Of the 2,248 doctors estimated to be overseas, it was estimated that at least 40 percent are permanently lost to Turkey because this proportion of doctors now in the United States have taken out licenses to practice. Based on recent trends it is estimated that there will be an annual loss of at least 90 doctors per year.

TABLE 8–2. DISTRIBUTION BY YEAR OF GRADUATION OF TURKISH DOCTORS ESTIMATED TO BE ABROAD, AS EXTRAPOLATED FROM 10 PERCENT SAMPLE SURVEY (1963)

Year of graduation	% from sample survey	Total living medical graduates	Total doctors abroad	Residual doctors in Turkey
Prior to 1940	6.1	1,550	137	1,413
1940–9	25.6	3,860	575	3,285
1950–9	60.0	4,840	1,350	3,490
1960–3	8.3	1,820	186	1,634
Totals	100.0	12,070	2,248	9,822[a]

[a]Addition of 188 Turkish graduates of foreign medical schools brings this up to slightly over 10,000, the figure used for total active doctors throughout this study.

Cumulative totals leading to the present supply of doctors are shown in Figure 8–1. The upper curve shows the total medical graduates; the second, the attrition from death with the main impact being in older graduates; and the lower curve, the loss of doctors overseas with the major effect being in graduates from the past fifteen years.

Projections

Calculations start with the 1964 base-line doctor population of 10,000. Three alternative projections were made (Figure 8–2).

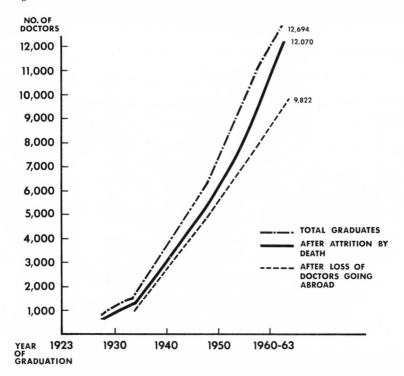

FIGURE 8–1. CUMULATIVE TOTALS OF TURKISH DOCTORS SHOWING TOTAL GRADU-
ATES SINCE 1923, MINUS THOSE WHO DIED AND THOSE OVERSEAS.

The first represents the net increment at present rates of production
and attrition. With 540 graduates per year reduced by 50 due to
death and retirement and 90 emigrating, the net increment is 400
doctors per year. Almost 5,000 doctors will be added by 1977 which
is half the present pool.

The second calculation takes into account the plans to build
five new medical schools. It is assumed that two of these will produce
100 doctors per year during the period 1972–7 with a net benefit
of 500 since these will probably not be subjected to serious attrition.

The third projection is based on the calculations presented in
Chapter 3 (pp. 111–13, 121), showing the great loss of medical
educational effort and resources because of dropouts and repeaters.
A loss equivalent to the output of two medical schools was calculated. The average increment of 200 doctors per year to be achieved
by remedying this situation by improved selection, education, and

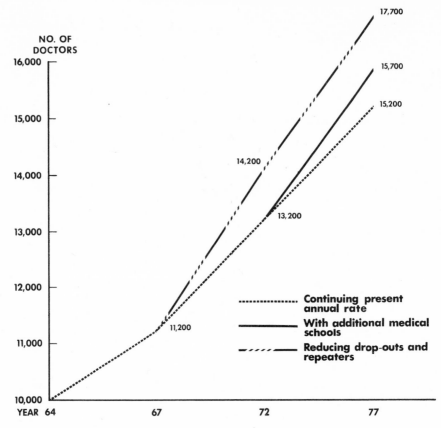

FIGURE 8-2. PROJECTIONS OF CUMULATIVE NUMBERS OF TURKISH DOCTORS BE-
YOND PRESENT ACTIVE NUMBER OF 10,000 (1964)—ALTERNATIVE INCREMENTS BY
ASSUMPTIONS BASED ON INCREASING GRADUATES AND REDUCING DROPOUTS AND
REPEATERS.

evaluation was estimated to start in 1968, which is optimistic because of the time needed to implement the required administrative
and educational reforms. The over-all increment over the ten-
year period represents an increase of two thousand doctors or one-
fifth of the present supply. It is apparent that the greatest immediate
acceleration of educational output will be achieved by an improvement in utilization of existing educational institutions.

PROJECTION OF SUPPLY OF TRAINED NURSING PERSONNEL

Trained nursing personnel are already in such short supply that
projections should be looked on primarily as a forward extrapolation of continuing shortages. Because of limitations in faculty and

poor utilization of present schools it has become apparent that a substantial increase in the supply of nurses can be achieved more readily by making better use of existing nursing schools than by opening new schools.

Registered Nurses

Since the shortage of registered nurses has been found to be greater than for any other category of health personnel, the basic assumption was made that the minimum rate of increase in nurse output should be equivalent to what Turkey has achieved in the past. In Figure 8–3, trend lines were drawn on a semilogarithmic scale showing the annual output of graduates since 1927 and the estimated cumulative increments to the national supply of *active* nurses. The total-supply curve was drawn on the basis of activity rates reported by a cross-section of graduates surveyed in 1964. These rates were applied uniformly to each cohort of graduates and the cumulative totals for each year were calculated. The straight line produced on the logarithmic scale lends itself readily to extrapolation. From an extension of this line the annual totals were read off to give minimum targets until 1977. Table 8–3 shows that the number of active female nurses will have to be more than tripled by 1977 to maintain the present rate of progress in increasing the nurse supply. Since only 62.5 percent of all graduates were found to be actively employed, the total number of graduates must be increased to allow for nurses not working. To get the required cumulative totals of graduates required, the annual output will have to go up from almost 500 in 1968 to an average annual production of 800 between 1973 and 1977.

In planning the necessary increase in nurse output it is usual to think mainly of opening new schools of nursing. This alternative was rejected for the next several years for the following reasons: (1) there are too few nurse teachers to staff new schools, even present schools have insufficient nurse teachers; (2) the investment in new facilities would be inordinate and unrealistic in view of the deficiencies in present schools; and (3) clinical facilities for practical teaching are particularly limited, although more use could be made of affiliation arrangements with existing hospitals such as those of social insurance.

A more realistic alternative is to make better use of existing schools. In Table 8–4 calculations are presented showing increased output based on the following goals to be achieved by 1977: (1)

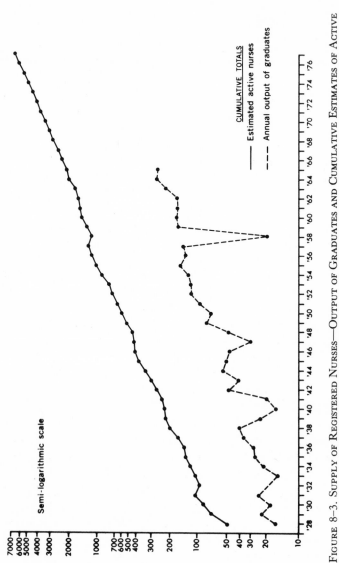

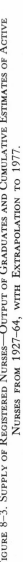

FIGURE 8–3. SUPPLY OF REGISTERED NURSES—OUTPUT OF GRADUATES AND CUMULATIVE ESTIMATES OF ACTIVE NURSES FROM 1927–64, WITH EXTRAPOLATION TO 1977.

TABLE 8–3. PROJECTED SUPPLY OF REGISTERED NURSES, USING CURRENT ANNUAL
RATE OF INCREASE AS STANDARD FOR PROJECTION AND INDICATING NUMBERS OF NEW
GRADUATES NEEDED ANNUALLY TO CONTINUE THIS RATE OF INCREASE

Years	Cumulative total no. of nurses expected to be active at end of time period (from Fig. 3)	Cumulative total no. of graduates required by end of time period (calculated from 62.5 percent activity rate)	Average no. of new graduates required annually
1964	1,852	2,963	258
1965–7	2,550	4,080	372
1968–72	4,100	6,560	496
1973–7	6,600	10,560	800

TABLE 8–4. PROJECTED SUPPLY OF FEMALE REGISTERED NURSES, ASSUMING FULL
USE OF EXISTING NURSING SCHOOLS, BY 1977

Years	Estimated supply of active nurses at end of period	Estimated cumulative total of graduates at end of period	Projected average annual output of new graduates per year		
			Ministry of health schools	Other schools	Total
1964	1,852	2,963	165	93	258
1965–7	2,696	4,313	310	140	450
1968–72	5,040	8,063	550	200	750
1973–7	8,008	12,813	650	300	950

the annual number of graduates from twelve existing lycee-level
schools of nursing which admit only one third or more females
should increase to fifty per school (this output has already been
achieved by some schools and appears to be an efficient level of
operation); (2) each of the eleven lycee-level health colleges which
admit mostly male students should average twenty-five female
graduates per year; and (3) each of the three university-level
nursing schools should increase its output to twenty-five nurses per
year from the present average of twelve per year.

These reasonable assumptions for improving utilization of nursing
schools would increase output by 1977 to more than meet the
requirements in Table 8–3, which used the same activity rate of

62.5 percent. In fact, there would be more than 1,400 additional active nurses which is about 75 percent of the total present, active supply.

An additional comment should be made on the danger that health colleges will be flooded by male candidates for training as *saglik memurus*, thus interfering with the proposed utilization of educational facilities for training female nurses (Table 8–5). A large number of male students in a health college tends to discourage female candidates for nursing. Also contributing significantly to their reluctance to attend is the lack of boarding facilities. Many more women go to exclusively female schools and to those where boarding arrangements are available. Schools such as the Red Crescent Nursing School in Istanbul, the Izmir Health College and the Maternity Hospital Health College in Ankara which meet these conditions have more than three times as many applicants as they can admit. By contrast, seven health colleges which do not provide boarding accommodations have 625 male students and only 37 females.

TABLE 8–5. STUDENT ENROLLMENT IN 1964–65 IN LYCEE-LEVEL HEALTH COLLEGES AND NURSING SCHOOLS, SHOWING MALE/FEMALE RATIOS RELATED TO THE AVAILABILITY OF BOARDING FACILITIES

Type of enrollment	Number of schools	Total enrollment	Average enrolled females per school	Male/ female ratio	Number of schools with boarding accommodation
Only female students in school	9	1,131	126	—	9
¹/₃ or more female students in school	3	474	54	2.0	3
Only male or mostly male students in school	11	1,646	15	10.0	4
Total	23	3,251	63	1.2	16

Another possibility is to attempt to increase nursing manpower by bringing inactive nurses back into nursing. Assuming an arbitrary activity rate of 80 percent rather than the present 62.5 percent, approximately 2,000 additional nurses would be available in 1977.

Although this is perhaps too ambitious a goal, there are many nurses who would work if appropriate arrangements could be made for reasonable hours and for positions in locations where their husbands are employed. The real value of making working conditions more attractive for nurses would be that recruitment would expand and produce a long-term increase in production and that quality would improve. More of the mature experienced nurses would continue to be available for supervision and teaching and thus help provide the needed faculty.

The combination, then, of better utilization of existing nursing schools plus better working conditions would substantially increase and improve the supply of active registered nurses. Both these changes appear necessary because adequate recruitment in order to get full utilization of schools will probably require more attractive working conditions for nurses.

Trained Nurses' Aides

As a result of the recent sharp increase in training programs for nurses' aides, there are fifty-one hospitals conducting courses in forty provinces with a total enrollment in 1964–5 of 997. Annual graduating classes averaged 19 per institution. The total number of graduates from 1955 to 1964 was 2,591. The average annual output of 259 will probably expand rapidly due to increased enrollment, especially with present plans to open health schools for training nurses' aides along with rural midwives.

The probable output from the present enrollment potential is calculated to be 665 graduates per year. By 1977 there should be more than five times the present number of graduates even with the present rate of production (Table 8–6). Since the course takes only two years and students are admitted after only five years of schooling, even more rapid expansion is possible. A large pool of potential recruits with only five years of schooling can be expected to be available.

Estimates for the supply of trained nurses' aides who would be active at the end of each time period were calculated on the assumption that 70 percent of the total graduates would be actively employed (Table 8–6). In 1964, 2,206 were reported by the Ministry of Health to be working. This is 85 percent of the graduates of nurses' aide training programs, but is probably an overstatement of the actual situation. The major source of error is the probability that some women are listed as nurses' aides on hospital records

TABLE 8–6. PROJECTIONS OF SUPPLY OF TRAINED NURSES' AIDES UP TO 1977, ASSUMING
THAT THE PRESENT ANNUAL OUTPUT WILL REMAIN CONSTANT[a]

Years	Estimated supply of active nurses' aides at end of period	Estimated cumulative total of graduates[a] at end of period
1964	2,206	2,591
1965–7	3,210	4,586
1968–72	5,538	7,911
1973–7	7,865	11,236

[a] 665 new nurses' aides is the estimated constant annual output used. This figure was calculated from a total enrollment of 997 in the eighteen-month assistant nurse training programs in 1964–5.

who have never graduated from a recognized training program. Because there is no system of licensure for nurses' aides and since we did not do a census, we were unable to check on these calculations.

To be used effectively, nurses' aides should not only be carefully trained but also they must be adequately supervised. It is here that the critical need for professional nurses is most acute. Hospitals which employ nurses' aides should have sufficient professional nursing staff to provide twenty-four-hour supervision. Each nurses' aide training course should have at least one professional nurse responsible for teaching and supervision of trainees.

Rural Midwives

The new nationalization and integration plans of the Ministry of Health will require many rural midwives for the rural health subunits. The rural midwife will also be a key figure in the new National Family-Planning Program.

A simple projection has been done (Table 8–7) showing increments of rural midwives as compared with urban midwives, based on the current production rate. The 2,543 trained midwives serving in rural areas for the Ministry of Health are only 55 percent of the 4,633 graduates of rural midwifery schools since 1938. This attrition rate of 45 percent obviously includes many midwives who have gone into private practice, especially in urban areas.

TABLE 8–7. PROJECTIONS OF SUPPLY OF RURAL AND URBAN MIDWIVES IN TURKEY
UP TO 1977

| | Estimated cumulative total of graduates | | |
Year	Rural midwives	Urban midwives	Total midwives
1964	3,104[a]	1,048[a]	4,152
1967	4,604[b]	1,348[c]	5,952
1972	7,104	1,848	8,952
1977	9,604	2,348	11,952

[a] Ministry of Health figures for midwives employed at end of 1964 in both urban and rural areas.

[b] About 500 graduates per year expected as village midwifery schools accelerate.

[c] Estimated 100 graduates per year from the three urban midwifery schools.

The increment rate for the projections was arbitrarily taken to be 500 per year graduating from rural midwifery schools. This is the net output of the present schools and has been projected merely to give a rough indication of the serious deficiency that is pending unless more schools are opened. Because of the high present attrition rates, either service conditions will have to be improved to keep midwives in villages or the output will have to be markedly increased to maintain the increment. The greatest deterrent to opening new schools is the lack of teaching staff, since even the present health schools are staffed by insufficient numbers of part-time teachers.

SUMMARY OF PROJECTED SUPPLY

Under existing conditions in Turkey, it has become evident that, in general, the best way of increasing health manpower is not to merely open more schools but to make better use of existing schools. Nursing schools and nurses' aides courses could accommodate many more students if proper boarding and other arrangements were made. Medical schools could improve output most readily by reducing dropouts and repeaters. Better teaching is essential and major curriculum modifications are needed to prepare all categories of personnel for the actual roles they are expected to fill. Finally, major improvements in services can be achieved by improving utilization of health personnel already trained.

9

PRESENT DEMAND FOR HEALTH MANPOWER

The demand estimates in this chapter are based as far as possible on actualities of presently available support plus the additional manpower needed to correct gross inequalities of distribution. Such estimates have greater practical relevance to present planning and policy decisions than theoretically sophisticated but often wishful ratios or norms borrowed from other countries. To be taken seriously, present demand data should represent openings for actual employment regardless of the numbers that professional judgment might suggest should be employed.

At the end of this chapter a summary brings together the various categories of health personnel for whom there seem to be immediate openings. Private practice demand has not been quantified but our information is summarized as general observations.

Most striking as evidence of the continuing pressure contributing to the present manpower imbalance is the finding that there are twice as many openings for doctors as for nurses—1,531 *vs.* 785. This is in spite of the fact that there are already more than five times as many doctors as nurses working in Turkey. When the demand for 679 midwives and 753 nurses' aides is added to the nurse demand, the total demand still comes to only 2,217.

CONCEPTUALIZATION

Most health manpower studies in the past have given only cursory attention to analyzing and projecting effective demand for health services. It is much easier to concentrate on the supply side of the equation. In general, demand estimates have been based on a series of accepted ratios such as doctors to population, other health workers to population, beds to population, or health personnel to hospital beds. These ratios have become recognized norms more through the accidents of chance development in particular countries than through any deliberate planning. Some open-market economic control has operated because numbers of health personnel tended to balance off at points where the general public was satisfied with the care they were receiving or were able to afford. The considerable differences which tended to appear in the more developed countries have been decreasing in recent years because ratios such as that of doctors-to-population have increasingly come to be status symbols in health development. Even Soviet planners initially derived their manpower standards from what satisfied spontaneous public demand and have tried to apply these standards as uniformly as possible in equalizing population ratios and work loads.

Although affluent countries have met most of their health needs through the operation of open-market economic controls, it has become increasingly evident that the planning efforts of most underdeveloped countries will require a different approach. The gap between demand and resources is so great that only a limited number of selected priority needs can be met. Manpower planning leads to deliberate efforts to stimulate the preparation of the most needed personnel. Frequently, difficult choices must be made between rational priorities and strong public desires based on national or professional pride.

The conceptualization of what economists refer to as the "demand side of the health manpower equation" then presents problems of special complexity. We have defined four approaches. The first is "biological need"—an approach based on professional judgment of the manpower needed to meet total health problems as determined by the best technical methods available. The classic example of an effort to measure demand in such terms is the Lee-Jones report[1] which attempted to calculate the manpower required to cope with the scientifically determined burden of disease in a U.S. population group according to standards set by expert professional judgment. Refined analyses of this kind have been only minimally useful. In any manpower study, however, some sort of initial definition of the health profile of a country is desirable in order to place priorities on the major disease problems and to identify those with special manpower requirements.

A second approach is to try to identify "popular desire" or the health services the people say they want. The many scientifically determined health problems about which people do not know or care will be left out of such an analysis. Conversely, the many manifestations of personal and community hypochondriasis which have no scientific basis will be included. One objective of health education is to minimize these discrepancies.

The third approach we have called "administratively and technically feasible demand." What can be done in health care is often much less than what should be done and the constraints are often not financial. The lack of technical knowledge or facilities is an obvious deficiency which cannot always be corrected by money. Oftentimes an even more important impediment to effective implementation of health programs is the lack of political and administrative machinery to provide the concentrated effort needed to achieve otherwise feasible and realistic goals.

The fourth approach we have termed "economic demand." Here monetary cost is the limiting factor. In an open-market economy people accept the reality that many of their physical complaints will remain untreated. Their own personal priorities may give precedence to alternative ways of spending money. In planned economies where priorities are supposed to be determined by social cost/benefit considerations, many health conditions are too expensive or too trivial to merit the cost of immediate attention and are deferred to an indefinite future. Usually, economic demand is the final determinant of health decisions in what economists have called "effective demand."

The coverage of these four approaches in Turkey in comparison with other countries is sketched impressionistically in a series of diagrammatic models (Figures 9–1, 9–2). Affluent countries tend to have considerable congruity of the areas covered by the squares representing the four approaches. They differ in that economic demand tends to follow biological need more in countries with centralized planning and socialized medicine, whereas it follows popular desire in countries with a large private sector. In Turkey there is a great discrepancy between biological need and popular desire on the one hand and the constraints of feasible demand and economic demand on the other. Since so much of health care is in the public sector, economic demand tends to follow biological need more than popular desire. The diagram for a grossly underdeveloped country suggests that the lack of congruity of the squares could almost be used as a measure of health development.

I Affluent country with large private sector

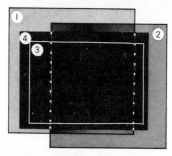

II Affluent country with socialized medicine and centralized planning

1. Biological Need
2. Popular Desire
3. Administratively & Technically Feasible Demand
4. Economic Demand

FIGURE 9–1. DIAGRAMMATIC MODELS OF RELATIONSHIPS BETWEEN BIOLOGICAL NEED, POPULAR DESIRE, ADMINISTRATIVELY AND TECHNICALLY FEASIBLE DEMAND, AND ECONOMIC DEMAND.

METHODOLOGY

Only minimal attention will be given to commonly accepted ratios for estimating present demand. Since part of the purpose of this study was to develop new methods of manpower analysis, a consistent effort has been made to try to develop more direct measures of demand. We have tried to distinguish between met and unmet demand. In terms of the above conceptualization, efforts to quantify demand have focused mainly on the third and fourth approaches dealing with "administratively and technically feasible demand" and "effective economic demand."

Unmet demand in institutions and organizations should be quantifiable by counting the unfilled, but budgeted, positions. The presumption seems reasonable that if a position is budgeted, then both administrative and economic demand exists. In Turkey, legal restrictions require that before a position can be budgeted funds

III Turkey

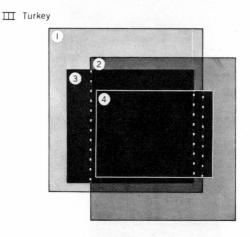

IV Country at early stage of economic development

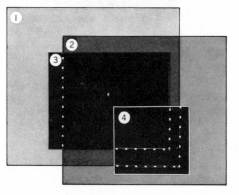

1. Biological Need
2. Popular Desire
3. Administratively & Technically Feasible Demand
4. Economic Demand

Figure 9–2. Diagrammatic Models of Relationships between Biological Need, Popular Desire, Administratively and Technically Feasible Demand, and Economic Demand.

must actually be available. This is different from some countries where, for political purposes, a large number of approved positions remain unfilled because there is no money in the budget to pay for them. In Turkey, however, another administrative maneuver has developed which complicates the data-gathering from official records. With positions actually budgeted, administrators are reluctant to let them remain unfilled even though appropriate staff are unavailable. Any individual available for any post at a specified salary level may, therefore, be assigned to any convenient opening, even though the position filled has no relationship to his actual work. These *ad hoc* designations tend to be retained indefinitely. There results a totally confusing mixture of budgeted positions which have little relevance to work performed. Clinicians are designated health officers, and teachers are filling administrators' posts; public health nurses hold positions created for teachers of basic science. Among Health Ministry auxiliaries the confusion is even greater. As an example of this administrative juggling, of the 988 budgeted positions for medical officers of health in 1964 only 619 were filled by such doctors, 277 positions were filled by clinical specialists working in hospitals, and 92 were vacant.

Data on unfilled positions presented in this analysis have been corrected for the above irregularities as far as possible. Much information was obtained from the institutional survey. An effort was made to get records of working positions filled rather than merely budgeted positions. In addition, the main calculation of unmet demand for hospital personnel was based simply on an effort to equalize the distribution of hospital beds by bringing all regions up to the minimum standard of 20 beds/10,000 population.

Quantifiable unmet demand exists mainly in hospitals and other institutions since they receive by far the largest investment of personnel and money. A disaggregated approach was used in this analysis with estimates for each system of health care being calculated separately in order to improve accuracy. Definition of particular areas with deficient facilities provided another basis for estimating the requirement for additional personnel. Because economic demand is the final determinant of effective demand, considerable effort was devoted to calculating costs in various types of institutions. The relative costs provide one basis for further estimating manpower utilization and the resources available for expansion.

PRODUCTIVITY OF DOCTORS

Any approach to understanding demand must start with appreciation of the fundamental principle that demand is for health services and not for manpower. Health services can usually be improved more effectively by increasing the utilization of personnel than by increasing numbers. Underlying most discussions about improving utilization of personnel is the basic theme of productivity. Great variations occur in the amount and quality of work accomplished by individuals who seem to have the same background and training. Even greater differences are found in the productivity of groups of people working in different systems and institutions. Individual differences in productivity are related mainly to strength of motivation and response to incentives. Group differences are more related to administrative factors and group incentives. Changes in productivity can be produced by the long-term process of molding motivation by education. More direct and short-range changes can be achieved by manipulating incentives and situational factors.

In the measurement of productivity in health activities, quantitative and qualitative considerations are equally important. In view of current recording inadequacies, it was difficult to get even relatively crude estimates of numbers of patient visits. Moreover, we not only wanted to know how many patients were seen, but also the quality of care received. Some individuals can do more in one patient contact than others can do in a dozen. Supporting services similarly modify output.

The productivity of all doctors in Turkey is low (Table 9–1). Calculations are presented as number of patients per doctor per year. This is an inadequate index but it has the advantage of simplicity. Data on public and private sector physicians were obtained from quite different sources. The data from the six government hospitals and two health centers which were included in the special survey of hospital costs described later were easily derived. The total number of patients seen in outpatient and inpatient services through the year was simply divided by the doctors on the staff. Specialists, general practitioners, and residents have specified hours of work which range from the specialists' six hours (three outpatient and three inpatient) to the residents' ten hours (three outpatient and seven inpatient). It did not add precision to try to derive hourly or daily productivity rate. The rate for private practitioners was derived from the average daily productivity rates recorded in the private-practice survey (Chapter 3, pp. 67–69). All doctors with private offices or clinics saw an average of 5.3 patients a day and full-time private practitioners saw 7.4 patients per day. Since private practitioners presumably put in as many work days a year as they can, we multiplied these figures by 300 days.

TABLE 9–1. COMPARISON OF DOCTOR PRODUCTIVITY IN PRIVATE SECTOR WITH PUBLIC SECTOR

	Patients seen per doctor per year		
	Outpatients	Inpatients	Total
6 government hospitals	1,800	200	2,000
2 health centers	3,200	300[c]	3,500
Total private sector	1,600[a]	—	1,600
Full-time private sector	2,200[b]	—	2,200
Mus Province before nationalization (1962)	1,300	130	1,430
Mus Province after nationalization (1963)	3,485	93	3,578

[a] Assuming maximum of 300 working days per year and an average of 5.3 patients per day.

[b] Assuming maximum of 300 working days per year and an average of 7.4 patients per day.

[c] Health center beds are occupied on a short-term basis, mostly for acute illnesses. The turnover is much higher than for hospital beds.

The productivity of government doctors is only a little greater than that of private practitioners. Health center doctors had the greatest productivity but this is still very low by international standards. It is true that 45 percent of doctors see patients in both public and private practice but even when the productivity averages for the two groups are added to give a maximum figure, the sum is only 3,400 patients per year. A particularly dramatic increase in productivity was observed as a result of the better organization in the nationalized health services. In the pilot year of work in Mus there was a two and a half times increase in patients seen per doctor over the previous year.

The public sector includes all health services performed by the Ministry of Health, other ministries (including Ministry of Defense), state economic enterprises, and Social Insurance. Except for the Ministry of Health, the others provide mainly curative health services for selected groups of persons. Activities were arbitrarily divided along administrative lines, even though some medical care agencies also provide public health services and vice versa. To simplify the classification, all health establishments which have hospital beds were defined as performing only medical care services.

Variations in Medical Care Services According to Supporting Agency

It proved impossible to get complete information about all health personnel working in public medical care services since the Ministry of Defense did not provide detailed information and one-fourth of the state economic enterprises' health institutions did not reply to repeated requests for data. Estimates have been made (Table 9–2) of the total number and type of health personnel in all institutions with the following adjustments for nonrespondent institutions: estimates of manpower in the Ministry of Defense were calculated from available data on number of beds in their institutions[2] and ratios of beds per type of health personnel derived from Ministry of Health institutions. This is undoubtedly an underestimate. For the nonrespondent institutions supported by state economic enterprises, calculations were merely an extrapolation based on the staffing patterns of institutions which did respond. The great variations in bed/personnel ratios suggest considerable unmet demand but do not permit precise calculation of numbers.

Cost of Hospital Services

No previous economic analyses of the costs of medical care services in Turkey have been made. There was, therefore, no standardized procedure for recording and collecting economic information in health institutions. The procedure for financing medical care services not only varies from agency to agency but each is complicated in itself. Few officials were aware of or interested in health economics.

To make a beginning, a few hospitals and health centers were selected for the cost-analysis study. The method of selection was far from random since it seemed more important to use institutions

TABLE 9–2. RATIOS OF BEDS PER EACH TYPE OF HEALTH PERSONNEL WORKING
IN PUBLIC MEDICAL CARE SERVICES BY SUPPORTING AGENCIES, TURKEY, 1964

Agencies	Number of beds per					
	Specialist	G.P. and resident	Pharmacist	Dentist	Nurse	Nurses' aide
Ministry of Health	25	82	1,495	555	54	29
Municipalities & local govt.	40	103	241	362	48	139
Other ministries & state economic enterprises	20	74	422	264	47	31
Social insurance (workers' insurance)	10	101	119	99	35	20
Average	22	70	55	34	50	30

Source: (a) For the Ministry of Health, municipalities, and local governments: The Ministry of Health's annual report on personnel for the year 1964 (un-published); (b) for other ministries, state economic enterprises, and social insurance institutions, our study data was collected through personal contact and questionnaires.

where good co-operation might be expected. From this study forms were developed which are now being used routinely on a trial basis to collect economic data in Ministry of Health institutions in eastern Anatolia. This should permit a more precise economic analysis in future studies.

The present observations do provide a preliminary notion of hospital costs. The selection of institutions was done by people familiar with the total medical and health structure of Turkey and a deliberate attempt was made to get representation of the existing range of expenditure and complexity. Of the five Ministry of Health and municipality hospitals selected, Ankara Hospital ranks near the top in money, personnel, and facilities available and the Corum Hospital ranks near the bottom. It is generally agreed that the two hospitals in Izmir fall in an intermediate position. The Izmir Chest Diseases Hospital represents the specialty chronic disease hospitals. Similar considerations were taken into account in choosing the hospitals supported by other agencies.

Since health centers tend to be essentially uniform in their level of expenditure, only two of the larger health centers were selected. Because they have somewhat greater bed capacity than the average health center, the cost per bed probably erred on the side of being an underestimate.

The selected hospitals proved to have approximately a 5 percent nonrandom sample of all hospital beds in Turkey. A validity check on the representativeness of the selected hospitals suggests, however, that the cost figures are probably an underestimate. Comparison of the ratio of beds to doctors and nurses in the selected hospitals as compared with all institutions with more than thirty beds seemed to be a useful index because nearly half of total hospital expenditures are for personnel. Table 9–3 shows that the selected hospitals had fewer personnel than the rest of the hospitals with particular deficiencies in nurses. This is partly due to the sampling error introduced by the fact that one-third of the total government beds were in the Izmir Tuberculosis Hospital where the personnel ratio is low, especially for nursing personnel. Our calculations, then, provide cost estimates which are conservative and minimal.

TABLE 9–3. COMPARISON OF NUMBER OF BEDS PER DOCTOR AND PER NURSE AND NURSE'S AIDE IN HOSPITALS SELECTED FOR THE COST STUDY AS COMPARED WITH ALL INSTITUTIONS WITH OVER THIRTY BEDS

	Number of beds per	
Group	Doctor	Nurse and nurses' aide
All institutions with over thirty beds	17	18
Selected hospitals	23	35

Detailed findings of hospital unit costs are shown in Table 9–4. The institutional data are averaged below:

Average cost *per patient day* in hospital = 45 TL ($5) Range: 23–92 TL

Average cost *per hospital bed per day* = 34 TL ($3.77) Range: 20–51TL

Average cost *per patient day* in health centers = 31 TL ($3.44) Range: 27–34 TL

Average cost *per hospital bed per day* in health centers = 12 TL ($1.33) Range: 10–16 TL

TABLE 9–4. HOSPITAL COSTS USED TO CALCULATE COST PER INPATIENT DAY AND PER HOSPITAL BED IN SELECTED PUBLIC INSTITUTIONS, FROM 1964 COST STUDY (TL)

Elements of cost (TL)[a]	Names of the institutions								
	Ankara State Hosp.	Ankara Railways' Hosp.	Corum State Hosp.	Izmir State Hosp.	Izmir[b] Municipality Hosp.	Izmir Social Insurance Hosp.	Izmir[b] Chest Diseases Hosp. (state)	Erban Health Center	Havza Health Center
Total cost per patient day	92	47	23	37	38	50	29	34	27
Personnel	36	34	9	17	20	28	12	16	18
Investment (Amortization)	8	4	2	2	3	5	2	4	3
Current Expenditure	47	19	11	17	14	17	15	14	6
Hospital occupancy rate	56	86	88	87	91	75	83	45	36
Cost per hospital bed	51	40	20	32	35	38	24	16	9

[a] 9 TL = 1 U.S. dollar.
[b] Excluding beds and personnel belonging to medical school of Izmir.

Few public sector hospitals serve the upper-economic group of the population. Since most hospitals fall in the middle-economic group, we used the average cost and the lowest cost for calculation of total expenditure on public medical care services. This was done so that any error would tend again to be an underestimate.

Figures on total patient days were unavailable for all public medical care services, but we did have the total number of beds and could calculate the over-all cost of hospital beds. The distribution of the annual costs of medical care services among different supporting agencies in the public sector is shown in Tables 9–5 and 9–6. Comparison of these figures with actual budgets can be made on a rough basis using the figures of the Ministry of Health. In 1964, the Ministry of Health requested 431,579,000 TL for medical care services but was given only 322,731,000 TL. In Table 9–5, the lowest estimated annual cost of medical care services of the Ministry of Health is 304,908,000 TL, which is only 18 million TL less than the actual expenditures. The average estimated annual cost, on the other hand, is 446,119,000 TL (Table 9–6) which is about 15 million TL more than the planned expenditures in 1964.

From this cost study, then, the annual cost of one hospital bed was estimated with a lower limit of 8,395 TL ($932) and an average cost of 12,410 TL ($1,378). Because of our deliberate

TABLE 9–5. ESTIMATED LOWEST ANNUAL COST OF PUBLIC MEDICAL CARE SERVICES PROVIDED BY SUPPORTING AGENCIES, FROM 1964 COST STUDY

Sponsoring agencies	No. of beds in		Annual lowest cost (× 1000 TL)		Total cost (× 1000 TL)
	Hospitals	Health ctrs. and other facilities	Hospitals	Health ctrs. and other facilities	
Ministry of Health	34,345	4,543	288,326	16,582	304,908
Municipalities and local government	2,497	1,123	20,963	4,099	25,062
Other ministries and state economic enterprises	15,174	1,687	127,386	6,158	133,544
Social insurance	4,134	42	34,705	153	34,858
Total	56,150	7,395	471,380	26,992	498,372

TABLE 9–6. ESTIMATED AVERAGE ANNUAL COST OF PUBLIC MEDICAL CARE SERVICES
PROVIDED BY SUPPORTING AGENCIES, FROM 1964 COST STUDY

Sponsoring agencies	No. of beds in		Annual average cost (× 1000 TL)		Total cost (× 1000 TL)
	Hospitals	Health ctrs. and other facilities	Hospitals	Health ctrs. and other facilities	
Ministry of Health	34,345	4,543	426,221	19,898	446,119
Municipalities and local government	2,497	1,123	30,988	4,919	35,907
Other ministries and state economic enterprises	15,174	1,687	188,309	7,389	195,638
Social insurance	4,134	42	51,303	184	51,487
Total	56,150	7,395	696,821	32,390	729,211

effort to use minimal figures, these figures are somewhat less than
the figures which had previously been used by the Ministry of
Health for its own planning estimates which were 15,410 TL
($1,712) in the Nationalized Health Service and 10,000 TL ($1,111)
outside the nationalized program.[3]

Regional Distribution of Hospital Services

An important element of demand analysis for public sector
services is the basic need to equalize regional distribution of health
services. The gross discrepancies in the regional bed/population
ratio are indicated in Table 9–7, with the range being from less
than 10 beds/10,000 population to over 50. These ratio variations
do not, however, match the ranking of the doctor/population
ratio, with the most marked difference being the relatively low
rank order of the bed ratio in southeastern Anatolia as compared
with eastern Anatolia where nationalization has started.

Calculation of Met and Unmet Demand for Hospital Beds

A basic policy decision which seems reasonable in the over-all
perspective of Turkey's general needs is that hospital services
should receive a relatively low priority in health planning. An
impressionistic ranking of expected cost/benefit returns suggests

TABLE 9-7. REGIONAL DISTRIBUTION OF HOSPITAL BEDS SUPPORTED BY PUBLIC
FUNDS, TURKEY, 1964

Statistical regions	No. of beds in			Midyear pop. (× 1000)	No. of beds per 10,000 population	No. doctors per 10,000 population
	Hospital	Health ctrs. and other facilities	Total			
Turkey in Europe[a]	14,781	1,529	16,310	3,006	54.3	13.1
Black Sea coast	4,379	953	5,332	4,907	10.9	1.1
Marmara and Aegean Sea coasts[a]	10,466	564	11,030	4,933	22.4	3.0
Mediterranean Sea coast	2,269	395	2,664	2,336	11.4	2.0
West Anatolia	4,886	753	5,639	2,590	21.8	1.5
Central Anatolia[a]	11,813	1,879	13,692	7,594	18.0	3.4
Southeast Anatolia	855	440	1,295	1,317	9.8	1.2
East Anatolia	6,701	882	7,583	3,946	19.2	1.1
Total	56,150	7,395	63,545	30,629	20.8	3.3

[a] University hospitals have an additional 3,510 beds divided as follows:

	No. beds	Total beds when added to above	Revised beds per population ratio
Turkey in Europe	1,110	17,420	57.9
Marmara and Aegean Sea coasts	671	11,701	23.7
Central Anatolia	1,729	15,421	20.3

the following priority listing: (1) preventive services, (2) ambulatory medical care, and (3) hospital services. Even with such a relatively low priority, however, a continuing investment in hospital facilities will be essential to provide a base for the rest of the health services.

Hospital services take up by far the largest proportion of the total health budget and total health manpower. Calculation of unmet demand for hospital services in the various regions of Turkey, therefore, represents the single most important economic component in the general health manpower distribution. Our basic analysis of unmet demand started with calculations based on data from the geographical regions presented in Tables 9–6 and 9–7. The regional distribution of the average annual cost of hospital services supported by public funds and the annual per capita expenditure on hospitals is shown in Table 9–8.

TABLE 9–8. REGIONAL DISTRIBUTION OF THE ESTIMATED AVERAGE ANNUAL COST OF TAX-SUPPORTED HOSPITAL SERVICES AND PER CAPITA EXPENDITURES, TURKEY, 1964

Statistical regions	Annual average cost of met demand ($\times$ 1,000 TL)	Midyear population ($\times$ 1,000)	Annual per capita expenditure (TL)
Turkey in Europe	190,130	3,006	63.25
Black Sea coast	58,517	4,907	11.92
Marmara and Aegean Sea coasts	132,353	4,933	26.83
Mediterranean Sea coast	29,888	2,336	12.79
West Anatolia	63,934	2,590	24.68
Central Anatolia	154,830	7,594	20.38
Southeast Anatolia	12,538	1,317	9.52
East Anatolia	87,022	3,946	22.05
Total	729,211	30,629	23.81

In attempting to achieve equalization of services, unmet demand for hospital services on a regional basis can be simply calculated by establishing a minimum standard. Since tax-supported hospitals are not dependent on open-market considerations of who can afford to pay for hospital services, the standard can presumably be set without primary regard to the socioeconomic status of the region. This is especially true since hospital services in Turkey are supported from central government financing. Such a simple administrative standard does not take into account the major variations in disease patterns around the country—but these usually have more relevance to preventive activities than to curative. The purpose of this calculation, then, is merely to estimate the cost of providing a minimum level of hospital services for each region.

The over-all average for Turkey is 20.8 hospital beds per 10,000 population. If the university hospital beds are included with the tax-supported hospital beds (Table 9–7), four of the eight regions of Turkey have more than 20 beds per 10,000 population. On this simple basis it seemed reasonable to establish twenty as the standard minimum figure for the calculation of unmet demand for hospital services. It is low by any international standard (Table 9–9), but is in accord with the higher priority accorded to preventive and ambulatory services.

TABLE 9–9. HOSPITAL BEDS PER POPULATION IN TWELVE OTHER COUNTRIES

Country	Year	Beds per 10,000
Turkey	1964	20
Ceylon	1959	33
Chile	1959	39
Czechoslovakia	1960	122
Israel	1960	59
Sweden	1959	111
U.S.	1960	92
England	1960	91
Denmark	1959	91
Yugoslavia	1957	45
U.S.S.R.	1960	82
Taiwan	1963	10
Peru	1964	24

Source: S. Btesh, "International Research in the Organization of Medical Care," Medical Care, Vol. 3 (1965), 1–41, except that Taiwan and Peru figures were from other Johns Hopkins manpower studies.

The regions of Turkey which fall below the hospital bed to population ratio of 20 per 10,000 tended to have a somewhat lower population density than the rest of Turkey and this reduced the total bed requirement. Table 9–10 shows the number of hospital beds necessary to bring the ratio up to twenty in these four regions. The total requirement of 8,138 hospital beds represents only a 13 percent increase above the present national total of 63,545 hospital beds supported by public funds.

The calculation is carried one step farther in Table 9–10 with estimates of the average and lowest annual costs of these additional beds. The average annual cost estimate for beds in these four regions was 100,000,000 TL ($11 million) and the lowest annual cost estimate was 68,318,000 TL ($7.5 million). In relation to the average annual cost of all present public hospital services (Table 9–8), the total increase required would add between one-seventh and one-tenth to present expenditures or a per capita annual increase for the country of 2–3 TL.

TABLE 9–10. UNMET MINIMUM DEMAND FOR HOSPITAL BEDS AND ANNUAL COST IN
FOUR REGIONS FALLING BELOW STANDARD OF 20 BEDS/10,000 POPULATION IN 1964

Statistical regions	Midyear population (× 1000)	No. of hospital beds			Annual coast (× 1000 TL)	
		Total no. beds needed	Met demand	Unmet demand	Lowest	Average
Black Sea coast	4,907	9,817	5,332	4,482	37,626	55,622
Mediterranean Sea coast	2,336	4,672	2,664	2,008	16,857	24,919
Southeast Anatolia	1,317	2,634	1,295	1,339	11,241	16,617
East Anatolia	2,946	7,895	7,583	309	2,594	3,835

On the basis of these calculations of unmet demand for hospital
beds, manpower requirements can be calculated (Table 9–11).
For simplicity, the present Ministry of Health staffing pattern
was used, not because it is ideal, but because it represents a practical
basis for equalizing services. It will require at least 322 specialists,
98 general practitioners, 5 pharmacists, 15 dentists, 150 nurses,
and 279 nurses' aides to bring hospital services to minimum standards.

TABLE 9–11. ESTIMATED MINIMAL UNMET DEMAND FOR HOSPITAL PERSONNEL IN FOUR
REGIONS FALLING BELOW STANDARDS OF 20 BEDS/10,000 POPULATION IN 1964

Statistical region	Unmet demand for hospital beds	Special-ists	General practi-tioners	Pharma-cists	Den-tists	Nurses	Nurses' aides
Ministry of Health standard of beds per personnel		25	82	1,495	555	54	29
Black Sea coast	4,482	179	54	3.0	8.0	82	153
Mediterranean Sea coast	2,008	80	24	1.0	4.0	37	69
Southeast Anatolia	1,339	54	16	0.9	2.0	25	46
East Anatolia	309	12	4	0.2	0.6	6	11

Demand calculations were based on the following corrections of the total number of budgeted positions in 1964 to get full-time equivalents of actual working personnel.

1. No unmet demand was found in the Central Organization of the Ministry of Health and the Central Hygiene Institute.

2. Since most medical officers of health working in health centers and maternal and child health centers also have their own private practices, two medical officers of health were considered to represent one full-time equivalent.

3. The total number of doctors working in administrative and public health services of municipalities and local governments was 345 in 1964. It was estimated that not more than 25 percent of their working hours were spent in these services. Most of them were appointed from among present health center physicians or medical officers of health who also had private offices. Only one-fourth of the number actually listed was, therefore, used.

4. For the tuberculosis, trachoma, leprosy, and syphilis control units, each doctor was considered to be full time if the unit was actually working, but the unit was considered active only if a doctor was employed.

5. Two of the existing regional hygiene institutes were considered equivalent to one full-time institute because of part-time employment.

6. For the cost study the estimates of annual per unit cost which were used were those which had previously been set up by the Ministry of Health for non-nationalized health services.[3]

Enquiry into the number and types of budgeted operating units which were actually working showed major deficiencies (Table 9–12). The greatest manpower deficiencies were in health officers' posts and the categorical programs for trachoma, MCH, and malaria. From these deficiencies of functioning administrative units, then, the actual manpower requirements for doctors were calculated as being 588 in 1964.

Table 9–13 shows the per unit distribution of budgeted costs among the various types of administrative and public health units according to Ministry of Health figures. It should be noted that 2.5 percent amortization for cost of buildings and 10 percent amortization for equipment, furniture, and motor vehicles were included in the current expenditure estimates.

TABLE 9–12. UNMET DEMAND FOR DOCTORS TO STAFF PUBLIC HEALTH
ADMINISTRATIVE UNITS IN TURKEY, 1964

Types of units	Total budgeted demand for administrative units	Unmet demand for administrative units	Percentage of met demand to total	Unmet demand for doctors
Central organization of the Ministry of Health	1	—	100	—
Directorates of health of the provinces	61	1	98	1
Office of the medical officer of health	591	271	54	271
Office of municipality and local government	230	146	37	146
Tuberculosis control dispensaries[a]	115	4	97	4
BCG vaccination teams	9	—	100	—
Mobile TB-screening teams	9	—	100	—
Trachoma control dispensaries	47	27	43	27
Leprosy control dispensaries	5	1	80	1
Syphilis control dispensaries	32	11	65	11
Dept. of malaria eradication[b]	28	13	54	78
MCH centers (with branches)	88	48	45	48
Central Institute of Hygiene	1	—	100	—
Regional hygiene institutes	2	1	50	1

[a] Fifty TB control dispensaries belonging to voluntary organizations are included, because they are mainly financed by the Ministry of Health.

[b] It is assumed that six doctors work in each department of malaria eradication.

Total annual expenditure can then be approximated according to met and unmet demand costs by multiplying the numbers of units in Table 9–12 by the costs per unit in Table 9–13. According to this calculation, 59 million TL out of the total budgeted amount of more than 212 million TL would have remained unspent. Allocated money which is not used is refunded to the government through the Ministry of Finance or spent for other purposes in

TABLE 9–13. ANNUAL COST OF VARIOUS TYPES OF ADMINISTRATIVE AND PUBLIC HEALTH UNITS ACCORDING TO BUDGETED STANDARDS OF MINISTRY OF HEALTH OUTSIDE OF NATIONALIZED HEALTH SERVICES IN 1964

Types of units	Personnel costs per unit (× 1,000 TL)	Other expenditure per unit (× 1,000 TL)	Total annual cost per unit (× 1,000 TL)
Central organization of the Ministry of Health	38,330	5,325	43,655
Dir. of Health of the Province	109	17	126
Office of med. officer of health	84	4	88
Office of municipality and local government	84	4	88
Tuberculosis control dispensaries	189	97	286
BCG vaccination teams	299	59	358
Mobile TB-screening teams	84	38	122
Trachoma control dispensaries	111	33	144
Leprosy control dispensaries	65	22	87
Syphilis control dispensaries	81	19	101
Dept. of malaria eradication	555	270	825
MCH	69	24	93
Central Institute of Hygiene	3,229	2,400	5,629
Regional hygiene institutes	651	300	951
Total	43,940	8,612	52,553

the Ministry of Health. Instead of the 212 million TL requested, the Ministry of Health was given almost 200 million TL in 1964. This indicates that the nonfunctioning units cannot be attributed to financial limitations because only 150 million TL would have been needed for all the functioning units. More probably the real reason they were not functioning was because of lack of manpower.

An accurate estimate of the regional distribution of unmet demand for public health services proved impossible to get. Data were available on the total number of public health units budgeted for each region but not on the units which were actually working. Calculations based only on the planned units were obviously biased to show more in the less developed regions than they actually had because that is where most of the nonworking units are located. Estimates were made differently for the following three categories of health activities:

1. Units which serve Turkey as a whole, e.g., Central Organization of the Ministry of Health, Central Institute of Hygiene, BCG

teams and mobile TB screening teams were equally distributed among the provinces. The calculations came out to 800,000 TL per province.

2. Units scattered all over the country, each serving a limited area, e.g., tuberculosis and syphilis control dispensaries, MCH centers, Department of Malaria Eradication, offices of health directors, medical officers of health, and municipality doctors, were assumed to have an even distribution of costs per unit and non-working unit. An average cost was obtained and multiplied by the number of units in the region.

3. Units established only in certain regions, and serving a limited area, e.g., trachoma and leprosy dispensaries and regional hygiene institutes, were assumed to be evenly distributed in those regions. Average unit costs were calculated just for these particular regions.

Even with the data biased to minimize discrepancies between regions, the expenditures on public health were particularly low in the less developed regions (Table 9–14). Per capita annual expenditures were consistently less than 5 TL in less developed regions.

TABLE 9–14. REGIONAL DISTRIBUTION OF THE COST OF ALL BUDGETED UNITS AND PER CAPITA EXPENDITURES FOR ADMINISTRATIVE AND PUBLIC HEALTH SERVICES IN TURKEY, 1964

Regions	Calculated annual cost of met demand (× 1000 TL)	Estimated midyear population (× 1000)	Per capita expenditure (TL)
Turkey in Europe	17,419	3,006	5.8
Black Sea coast	21,927	4,907	4.5
Marmara and Aegean Sea coasts	26,813	4,933	5.4
Mediterranean Sea coast	11,947	2,336	5.1
West Anatolia	15,649	2,590	6.0
Central Anatolia	33,510	7,594	4.4
Southeast Anatolia	6,364	1,317	4.8
East Anatolia[a]	17,228	3,946	4.4
Total	150,857	30,629	4.9

[a] The special regional units in the nationalized health services areas are not included.

One reason why manpower deficiencies could not be calculated by regions was because of the larger number of individuals who hold multiple jobs in the less developed regions. Also, since positions in the Ministry of Health are often assigned without regard to officially budgeted positions, many health personnel who are supposed to be working in the less developed provinces are actually filling positions in places of their choice. The regional maldistribution is, therefore, certainly worse than above calculations show.

NATIONALIZED HEALTH SERVICES

By 1964, the nationalized health services had been started in six provinces—Mus, Hakkari, Van, Agri, Bitlis, and Kars—representing 5 percent of the total population of Turkey. In addition to previously existing hospitals, 126 health units had been established. The manpower required to meet the standards of the nationalized health services has already been described. Table 9–15 shows the progress in meeting these standards in the six provinces where nationalization of health services had been started by 1964. The planned services and personnel requirements for these standards are designated as total demand and available services and personnel as met demand. Percentages of those actually

TABLE 9–15. PROGRESS IN FILLING PLANNED POSITIONS IN THE NATIONALIZED HEALTH SERVICES IN SIX PROVINCES IN TURKEY, 1964

Units of the Services	Met demand	Unmet demand	Total demand	Percentage of met to total demand
Health unit	126	47	173	73
Hospital bed	710	790	1,500	47
Specialist	67	72	139	48
General practitioner	150	82	232	65
Pharmacist	5	9	14	36
Dentist	11	4	15	73
University-level trained health personnel	9	3	12	75
Saglik memuru	271	18	289	94
Nurse	89	153	242	37
Nurse's aide	103	5	103	95
Village midwife	321	326	647	50

working range from 37 percent for nurses to 95 percent for *saglik memurus* and nurses' aides. The percentage for general practitioners was 65 percent and for specialists almost 50 percent.

To calculate the annual cost of the nationalized health services in these six provinces, the figures provided by the Ministry of Health were used (Table 9–16). We were not able to obtain data on actual expenditure. The cost of personnel was not separated out. The striking feature is the relatively greater expenditure on health units than hospitals.

TABLE 9–16. ESTIMATED ANNUAL COST OF MET AND UNMET DEMAND IN SIX PROVINCES WITH NATIONALIZED HEALTH SERVICES IN TURKEY, 1964

| Units of the Services | No. existing in 1964 | Annual cost of ($\times$ 1000 TL) | | | |
		Per unit	Met demand	Unmet demand	Total demand
Health units[a]	126	180	22,680	8,460	31,140
Hospitals[b]	7	1,541	10,787	12,328	23,115
Provincial health dir.	6	330	1,980	—	1,980
Dept. of MCH	5	68	340	68	408
Dept. of malaria eradication	6	868	5,208	—	5,208
TB control dispensary	6	395	2,370	—	2,370
Trachoma dispensary	4	198	792	396	1,188
Leprosy and VD dispensary	5	141	705	141	846
Total			44,862	21,393	66,255

[a] All the existing health units were considered rural.

[b] Available number of beds was 710 in twelve hospitals. The figures used are equivalent to seven hospitals with 100 beds each.

EDUCATIONAL INSTITUTIONS

Training institutions for health personnel must increase their own teaching staff to meet future manpower needs, thus generating a further manpower demand. The Ministry of Health has given special emphasis to educational institutions since 1960, but a great unmet demand remains, requiring both quantitative and qualitative improvement.

1. There is great popular demand for more university-level institutions. In fact, however, the immediate need is not so much

for an increase in the number of institutions as for the provision of qualified and effective teachers for existing institutions. Our estimates are that there is at least a 50 percent unmet demand in the number of university-level faculty. As an example of the severe shortage, almost all the teachers at the private dentistry and pharmacy schools are also permanent staff members of the dentistry and pharmacy schools of Istanbul University. Some teach in Ankara University as well.

2. In 1964 there were 80 part-time doctors, 73 nurses, and 119 other full-time teaching staff in the twenty health colleges and three nursing schools actively providing lycee-level training. This gives a ratio of 44 students per nurse and 41 students per part-time doctor.

3. In the middle-school-level health schools for rural midwives the shortages were even greater with 61 students per nurse and per part-time doctor. Only a small fraction of the teachers represented the occupational group being trained with a ratio of 529 students per midwife.

No teachers were provided for nurses' aides courses, since the hospital staff assumed responsibility for operating these courses along with their usual service responsibilities.

PRIVATE SECTOR

Institutional Services

Unfortunately, we were not able to collect much information about the number and type of personnel working in private institutions. Only forty of the seventy-six hospitals surveyed gave complete information. Detailed personnel lists collected from these forty hospitals are summarized in Table 9–17.

The special study on the cost of medical care included three private hospitals. Detailed findings on the unit cost in private hospitals showed a remarkable range of variation (Table 9–18). Doctors' fees were not included but were estimated to be an additional 10 TL per day per hospital bed as compared with about 4 TL per day in Ministry of Health hospitals.

The variation in daily cost per hospital bed in these private hospitals was not unexpected since the three were selected specifically to provide a wide range. The Admiral Bristol Hospital is exceptional in its clientele and cost. To obtain figures more readily comparable with other Turkish hospitals, the average bed cost of the other two hospitals was computed and 10 TL per bed for

TABLE 9–17. NUMBER AND TYPES OF HEALTH PERSONNEL WORKING IN FORTY
PRIVATE HOSPITALS IN TURKEY, 1964
(TOTAL NUMBER OF BEDS = 2,119)

Type of personnel	No. of personnel	Ratio of beds per personnel	Av. personnel per private hospital
Specialists	128	17	3.2
General practitioners and residents	30	71	0.8
Pharmacists	10	212	0.2
Dentists	5	424	0.1
Nurses and nurses' aides	142	15	3.5
Total	315	7	

TABLE 9–18. UNIT COST PER PATIENT DAY AND PER HOSPITAL BED IN THREE
SELECTED INSTITUTIONS SUPPORTED BY PRIVATE AGENCIES

Elements of the costs (TL)	Private hospitals		
	Izmir, Konak Clinic	Istanbul, Admiral Bristol Hospital	Istanbul, Armenian Hospital
Personnel Cost	26.97	68.70	8.56
Investment (amortization)	28.84	22.09	3.60
Current expenditure	47.55	79.30	8.05
Unit cost per patient day	103.36	170.09	20.21
Hospital occupancy rate (%)	40.00	79.00	61.00
Unit cost per hosp. bed	41.35	134.30	12.33

doctors' fees was added to obtain a rather conservative average daily cost. One hospital bed in the private sector thus was estimated to cost 37 TL per day as compared with 34 TL in Ministry of Health hospitals. This standard unit cost was multiplied by beds to estimate the annual cost of private hospital services with the total coming to more than 100 million TL (Table 9–19).

The regional distribution of private medical care services shows a strictly urban localization being limited largely to the Istanbul area with some beds in Hakkari and Izmir (Table 9–20). The regional discrepancy is shown most dramatically when per capita

TABLE 9–19. ESTIMATED AVERAGE ANNUAL COST OF PRIVATE HOSPITAL SERVICES BY
SUPPORTING AGENCIES IN TURKEY, 1964
(ANNUAL COST OF ONE BED: 37 TL × 365 DAYS = 13,505 TL)

Sponsoring agencies	Number of beds	Total annual cost (× 1000 TL)
Proprietary institutions	1,573	21,243
Business and industry	194	2,619
Philanthropic organizations	5,684	76,762
Total	7,451	100,624

TABLE 9–20. REGIONAL DISTRIBUTION OF PRIVATE HOSPITAL SERVICES WITH AVERAGE
ANNUAL COST, TURKEY, 1964

Regions	No. of beds	Total annual average cost (× 1000 TL)	Annual per capita cost (TL)
Turkey in Europe	4,082	55,127	18.3
Black Sea coast	210	2,836	0.6
Marmara and Aegean Sea coasts	1,000	13,505	2.7
Mediterranean Sea coast	381	5,145	2.2
West Anatolia	212	2,863	1.1
Central Anatolia	1,186	16,016	2.1
Southeast Anatolia	209	2,823	2.1
East Anatolia	171	2,309	0.6
Total	7,451	100,624	3.3

cost is calculated. The Istanbul area annual per capita cost was
over 18 TL, whereas each of the other regions was only 1–2 TL per
year.

Private Practice

Quantification of unmet demand in the private sector has been
largely a process of trying to identify "soft spots" that market
economic adjustments have not equalized. The correlation between
per capita income of the general population and total number of
doctors by region was calculated to see how the distribution of
physicians responds to available money. The rank orders shown in
Table 9–21 produce a significantly high correlation coefficient,

TABLE 9-21. RELATION BETWEEN PER CAPITA GNP AND POPULATION/DOCTOR
RATIO IN TURKEY

| Regions | Per capita GNP in 1960 (TL) | No. of persons per doctor in 1964 | Rank order | |
			GNP	Pop.–Doctor Ratio
Turkey in Europe	2,645	761	1	1
Black Sea coast	1,212	8,841	8	8
Marmara and Aegean Sea coasts	1,677	3,373	3	3
Mediterranean Sea coast	1,531	4,938	5	4
West Anatolia	1,786	6,623	2	5
Central Anatolia	1,579	2,965	4	2
Southeast Anatolia	1,306	8,284	6	6
East Anatolia	1,217	8,749	7	7
Average	1,594	3,063	—	—

$R = 0.83$. Per capita GNP was calculated from the only available official calculations (1960) and population per doctor ratio was taken from our survey data in the doctors' census.

About 11 percent of the doctors living in Turkey were in full-time private practice in 1964. Another 48 percent had private offices or clinics in addition to regular employment in the public sector and were classified as part-time private doctors, the remaining 40 percent were in full-time public service. It is clear from Table 9-22 that there is a general similarity in the regional distribution of doctors. The major difference is that in Central Anatolia where the capital city is situated, many doctors work directly for the central government and this leaves a smaller percentage of doctors on public support to be distributed in the other regions.

A preliminary indication of unmet demand in the private sector may be the proportion of doctors in part-time private practice. They do not feel secure enough in private practice to go into it full time. On the other hand, with the relative security of a public position they find that they can earn adequate money in the more lucrative private sector. Presumably as economic conditions improve sufficiently to make private practice more secure, urban physicians may leave their less lucrative government posts.

TABLE 9–22. REGIONAL DISTRIBUTION OF SALARIED GOVERNMENT, PRIVATE, PART-TIME PRIVATE DOCTORS IN TURKEY, 1964

Statistical regions	Total no. of doctors	% distr. of total doctors	% distr. of public doctors	% distr. of part-time private doctors	% distr. of private doctors	% distr. of population of Turkey
Turkey in Europe	367	37.1	38.3	36.1	37.3	9.8
Black Sea coast	51	5.2	2.0	7.4	6.0	16.0
Marmara and Aegean Sea coasts	137	13.9	8.9	16.0	22.0	16.1
Mediterranean Sea coast	54	5.5	2.8	6.1	11.9	7.6
West Anatolia	30	3.0	1.0	5.0	1.7	8.5
Central Anatolia	274	27.7	39.6	20.6	16.9	24.8
Southeast Anatolia	19	1.9	1.8	2.3	0.9	4.3
East Anatolia	56	5.7	5.6	6.5	2.5	12.9
Total No.	988		394	476	118	
Percent		100.0	39.9	48.2	11.9	

The full-time practitioners probably represent a solid commitment to private practice. The percentage distribution of private practitioners in comparison with public physicians shows a clear economic influence. In the relatively more affluent regions of Marmara and the Mediterranean the percentage of private physicians was almost twice the public. On most of the Anatolian plateau the distribution was essentially reversed.

SUMMARY OF PRESENT UNMET DEMAND

As a preliminary indication of unmet demand in the public sector, it seemed reasonable to simply add up vacancies in budgeted positions and the gross deficiencies calculated in this chapter (Table 9–23). Efforts to arrive at such totals are tentative and hazardous. The major immediate shortages are for general practitioners 1,137, specialists 394, nurses 785, midwives 679, and nurses' aides 753. These cumulative totals are derived from subcalculations of unmet demand for administrative and public health positions (Table 9–12), the nationalized health services (Table 9–15), plus appropriate government records of unfilled positions. These figures are undoubtedly understatements. Data on nurses are particularly fragmentary. Until the role and contribution of the nurse are more generally recognized, there is no prospect that adequate employment opportunities will be created.

The estimates of unmet demand in the private sector led to generalizations rather than specific numerical data. In general, however, it seems clear that private sector demand is essentially saturated. The present 10 percent of doctors who are full-time private practitioners represent the solid core of private practice. Almost half of all doctors are in part-time private practice but are not particularly happy with the arrangement.

The following generalizations seem justified:

1. There is little unmet demand for specialists. There are more openings for general practitioners, especially to staff health centers. Pharmacist, dentist, and to a lesser extent, *saglik memuru* vacancies in government services have been for the most part filled.

2. Shortages of nursing and midwifery personnel are much greater than the calculations show. Presently recognized demand is mainly in the nationalized health services. The simple statistic that there are only 1.8 registered nurses per medical institution shows the severity of the shortage. Even more dramatic is the

TABLE 9–23. PRESENT DEMAND SUMMARY, CUMULATIVE NUMBERS OF PERSONNEL
NEEDED IN TURKEY, 1964

	Existing Ministry of Health vacancies[a]	Estimated deficiencies in public sector hospitals for 4 regions[b]	Nation- alized services[c]	Nursing insti- tutions	Total
All doctors					1,531
Specialists	—	322	72	—	394
General practitioners	957	98	82	—	1,137
Pharmacists	100	5	9	—	114
Dentists	13	15	4	—	32
Saglik memurus	325	—	18	—	343
Midwives	276	—	326	77	679
Nurses	300	150	153	172[d]	785
Nurses' aides	469	279	5	—	753

[a] 588 doctors required based on unmet demand for existing public health units, refer to Table 9–12. 369 doctors required to fill budgeted positions in health centers, refer to data showing 988 budgeted positions but only 619 positions filled. Rest of data taken from Ministry of Health's list of unfilled positions.

[b] Based on manpower needed to meet unmet demand for hospital beds in the four regions falling below a standard of 20 beds per 10,000, refer to Table 9–11.

[c] Based on unmet demand in nationalized services in 1964, refer to Table 9–15.

[d] Standards for nurse-teacher to student ratio and midwife-teacher to student ratio of 1:20 students were used as recommended by the Turkish Government in the "Overview of Nursing in Turkey," CENTO *Conference of Nursing Education* (Teheran, 1964), pp. 155.

finding that there are more than five doctors for every nurse in Turkey.

3. In this chapter several different efforts have been made to initiate more sophisticated attempts to measure economic demand. Data have been collected on the cost of various types of medical services. In general, the estimates seem reasonable and in keeping with Turkish resources. They also show that hospital services are as expensive relative to other health services as anywhere else in the world. On a cost basis this supports the general conclusion that priority given to preventive and ambulatory services will bring greater health returns for less investment. More precise cost/benefit analyses will have to wait until better methods of measuring health benefit have been developed.

REFERENCES

1. R. I. Lee and L. W. Jones, *The Fundamentals of Good Medical Care* (Chicago: University of Chicago Press, 1933).
2. Dr. Feridun Frik, *Cumhuriyet Deuri Saglik Mizmetleri*, 1923–63 (Turkey, 1964).
3. *Expenditures Necessary for the Nationalization of Health Services and the Finance of the Project*, Publication No. 14 (Ankara School of Public Health, 1965).

10

PROJECTION OF DEMAND

Projecting demand into the future is even more speculative than defining present demand. However, it is essential to manpower planning and it provides a better basis for determining educational requirements than any other method.

Turkey's present shortage and imbalance of health manpower will become progressively worse if appropriate action is not taken. Demand will be increased by the continuing high population growth rate of about 3 percent per year, expanded use of medical and hospital services, and a changing pattern of medical practice resulting from the nationalization of health services.

ALTERNATIVE METHODS OF PROJECTING DEMAND

Demand projections must be conditional since uncertainties exceed any mathematically definable expectations. Only by defining a specific set of conditions does it become possible to extrapolate present trends to the future while allowing for modifying variables within a limited range of accuracy and time. To provide a reasonable basis for policy decision, it is appropriate to define several different sets of conditions with alternative projections relevant to each. For alternative projections to be useful for policymakers and administrators, these conditions should be stated in terms of the major administrative choices available. The final projections should be placed in a range from minimum to maximum reasonable requirements.

Present conditions in Turkey suggested three methods of projecting manpower demand: (1) the minimum projections based on proportional increase of personnel to maintain the 1962 population/manpower ratio, (2) the Ministry of Health's plans for nationalized health services and integrated services, plus a continuing private sector, (3) the maximum projections based on an adaptation of the manpower standards set by the WHO Conference on Medical Education for the eastern Mediterranean region in 1962. The population/personnel ratios used as bases for the three alternative projections vary considerably as shown in Table 10–1.

TABLE 10–1. POPULATION/PERSONNEL RATIO ACCORDING TO FOUR ALTERNATIVE BASES FOR PROJECTIONS

Type of personnel	1962 population personnel ratio	Nationalized plan[a] (rural & urban)	Integrated plan	Payzin-Tekesin
No. of persons per each type of health personnel				
Specialist	4,358	10,000	—	2,000
General practitioner	10,682	10,000	37,500	
Pharmacist	19,506	100,000	—	10,000
Dentist	18,965	100,000	—	10,000
Saglik memuru	8,538	10,000	6,250	—
Midwife	7,883	3,333	1,875	—
Nurse	17,794	6,667	—	5,000
Nurse's aide	—	14,285	—	—
Hospital beds	395	500	—	—

[a] Additional provincial health personnel listed in Chapter 9 were not included in these calculations because the sizes of populations served varied according to the size of the provinces.

Minimum Projection to Meet the Population Increase

The inadequate ratios of population to manpower in 1962 were used for the minimum projections. The national population increase between 1955 and 1960 was at the rate of 2.9 percent per year. Projections were based on average annual rates of growth by provinces applied to the manpower available in each province. Since 1963 was the first year of the nationalization plan, 1962 was taken as the starting year for the projections. This had the advantage that the calculated projections for 1964 could be checked against the actual findings of our survey. The figures were encouragingly close. In the present scarcity situation, it is neither reasonable nor politically wise to plan for no improvement in the over-all manpower ratio. These calculations are useful mainly as a base line to be applied to specific categories of personnel. As priority decisions are made that certain categories need immediate expansion while others are less urgently needed, the base line provides the minimum level of production needed to prevent a deteriorating ratio in low priority categories. These minimum figures cover both public and private sectors. The two governmental plan projections, to be presented next, estimate the additional public sector expansion needed to achieve both regional equalization and an appropriate increase of the most needed categories of health workers.

Ministry of Health Plans

Nationalization Health Services Plan. The following standards have been established to serve one rural-type health unit with 7,000–10,000 population (10,000 is used in these calculations because with the expected population increase this figure will be reached in the present units in about twelve years). In every rural health unit the government will support at least: one general practitioner, one *saglik memuru*, one nurse, and three village midwives, while in urban health centers the ratio will be the same with twice this number of staff for double the population.

As a start, one hospital with 100 beds is planned for 100,000 persons. Future plans call for 200 beds for every 100,000 population (20 beds per 10,000) which was the ratio used as a minimum standard in Chapter 9 to calculate present unmet demand. The hospital will serve both rural and urban populations. Each 100,000 population unit is to have ten specialists for the hospital plus one pharmacist, one dentist, five hospital nurses, and seven nurses' aides.

Comparison of the columns in Table 10–1 shows that the nationalized health service standards appear to be lower for some categories of health manpower than those now active. For instance, there are already twice as many specialists as the nationalized plan requires. This apparent discrepancy is spurious since the nationalized plan is additive in its manpower demand to the existing private sector supply. It will be absorbing an unknown fraction of present manpower and gaining a large part of needed recruits as they graduate. The nationalization plan will increase the balance of manpower in the public sector, especially in the less developed provinces.

Integrated Health Service Plan. An interim plan was developed by the Ministry of Health for provinces in which malaria eradication programs were ready for the surveillance phase and therefore would need a health infrastructure to carry on the work. The program mainly requires auxiliaries since doctors work in a supervisory role. According to the plans each unit of 37,500 population will have one practitioner, six *saglik memurus* (1 per 6,250), and thirty midwives (1 midwife per 1,875 or almost twice as many as in the nationalized plan). Projections for the integrated plan are shown only for 1972 since the malaria program will require these services by then. Only those provinces which are not scheduled to have nationalization coverage are included. If both plans are deferred as now seems likely projections will merely be postponed.

Maximum Projections According to Payzin-Tekesin

Maximum projections were based on standards for health manpower which had been set by the WHO Conference on Medical Education, eastern Mediterranean region, Teheran, in 1962. These were adapted for Turkey by Dr. Sabahattin Payzin, Professor of Microbiology, School of Medicine, Ankara University, and Dr. Ali Tekesin, Assistant Director General of Education, Ministry of Health and Social Welfare. The personnel to population ratios are 1 physician per 2,000 population, 1 dentist and 1 pharmacist per 10,000 population, 1 nurse per 5,000 population.

DEMAND PROJECTIONS FOR SPECIFIC CATEGORIES OF MANPOWER AND HOSPITAL BEDS

Specialists

To maintain the present ratios a steady increase is necessary (Table 10–2). The 1964 projection of 7,255 specialists compares with the estimated figure of 7,350 obtained from the doctors' census. Calculations in Chapter 9 show relatively little present unmet demand for specialists. With the continuing general expansion of hospital training facilities to meet their own staffing needs (Chapter 3, p. 55) there is every indication that future supply of specialists will continue to increase faster than present standards of demand. The nationalization plan's demand for specialists will expand also but the numbers will be small. In 1977 they will represent less than one-fourth of all specialists.

TABLE 10–2. CUMULATIVE PROJECTED DEMAND FOR SPECIALISTS (1962–77)

Year	Estimated[a] population	To maintain 1962 population/ personnel ratio	National- ization plan	Payzin- Tekesin (all doctors)
1962	29,362,000	6,746	—	14,696
1964	31,138,000	7,255	151	—
1967	33,962,000	8,096	652	17,033
1972	39,298,000	9,729	1,312	19,563
1977	45,542,000	11,707	3,989[b]	22,656

[a] Population size was estimated by projecting the growth rates by province and then totaling. The results differ slightly from projections based on total population.

[b] Urban nationalization requirements were subtracted for Ankara, Istanbul, and Izmir for 1977 to allow for probable use of available personnel.

Maximum projections based on Payzin-Tekesin standards were calculated only for all doctors, so that it is impossible to separate specialists from general practitioners. The 1964 number should be doubled to meet the 1977 target of 22,656 doctors.

General Practitioners

Less than one-third of present Turkish doctors are general practitioners. The strong movement toward specialization within the profession will make it increasingly difficult to maintain present ratios (Table 10–3). The nationalization plan will create a growing

TABLE 10–3. CUMULATIVE PROJECTED DEMAND FOR GENERAL PRACTITIONERS (1962–77)

Year	To maintain 1962 population/ personnel ratio	Ministry plans		Total
		Nationalized services	Integrated services	
1962	2,752	—	—	—
1964	2,947	151	—	151
1967	3,268	652	—	652
1972	3,889	1,312	240	1,552
1977	4,635	4,070[a]	—	4,070

[a] Urban nationalization requirements were subtracted for Ankara, Istanbul, and Izmir for 1977 to allow for probable use of available personnel.

demand for general practitioners. Most of these will probably
come from recent medical school graduates. By 1977 almost half of
all general practitioners should be in the nationalized health services, according to forward projections of present ratios.

Pharmacists and Dentists

Present pharmacist to population ratios will presumably be
required to meet private sector demands (Table 10–4). The requirements of the nationalized services are not great. The maximum
projections, however, would require doubling the present supply.

TABLE 10–4. CUMULATIVE PROJECTED DEMAND FOR PHARMACISTS AND DENTISTS
(1962–77)

Year	To maintain 1962 population/personnel ratio		Nationalization plan	Payzin-Tekesin
	Pharmacists	Dentists	Pharmacists and dentists	Pharmacists and dentists
1962	1,507	1,550	—	2,939
1964	1,615	1,664	14	—
1967	1,794	1,852	65	2,405
1972	2,138	2,215	141	3,928
1977	2,553	2,654	398[a]	4,531

[a] Urban nationalization requirements were subtracted for Ankara, Istanbul,
and Izmir for 1977 to allow for probable use of available personnel.

The projected demand for dentists approximately equals that for
pharmacists. It is apparent that dental care receives lower priority
than medical care generally and that dentist services will continue
to concentrate on the urban private sector. Some type of dental
auxiliary is needed in rural areas but no plans have been developed.

Saglik Memurus and Midwives

Both of the new public sector plans rely heavily on *saglik memurus*
for many important preventive functions. With appropriate incentives many of those now employed in both public and private
work will transfer to the health services.

The projected demand for midwives slightly exceeds that for
saglik memurus (Table 10–5). The new nationalization and integration plans will certainly produce a marked expansion of demand

for rural midwives to staff the rapidly developing maternal and child health services. They will also undoubtedly play an important role in the new National Family-Planning Services. These sharply increasing figures must be considered minimum demands and a massive effort will be needed to expand the output from health schools.

TABLE 10–5. CUMULATIVE PROJECTED DEMAND FOR *Saglik Memurus* AND MIDWIVES[a] (1962–77)

Year	To maintain 1962 population/personnel ratio		Nationalization plan		Integrated plan (rural areas)	
	Saglik memurus	Midwives	*Saglik memurus*	Midwives	*Saglik memurus*	Midwives
1962	3,443	3,729	—	—	—	—
1964	3,647	3,948	151	452	—	—
1967	3,797	4,302	652	1,950	—	—
1972	4,605	4,970	1,403	4,346	1,450	4,832
1977	5,339	5,752	3,989	11,970[b]	—	—

[a] Includes midwives trained for urban areas as well as those trained for rural areas.

[b] Urban nationalization requirements were subtracted for Ankara, Istanbul, and Izmir for 1977 to allow for probable use of available personnel.

Nurses

It has been reiterated that the need for nurses in Turkey is greater than for any other category of personnel. The calculations show, however, a relatively modest demand (Table 10–6). The increase of nurses, in fact, exceeded the minimum projected demand in 1964 (1,676); the actual supply was 1,852. Because the present great need is felt most acutely in hospital nursing, an additional calculation has been included to show what would be required to improve hospital nursing standards. The present ratio is approximately forty hospital beds per nurse. If this ratio were reduced to twenty beds per nurse which is the standard accepted for the nationalization plan, then the number of hospital nurses would obviously have to be doubled. If projected demand for nurses in hospitals were met, there would be three to four nurses per institution instead of the present average of less than two nurses per institution, thus permitting twenty-four-hour coverage. Approximately

TABLE 10–6. CUMULATIVE DEMAND PROJECTION FOR NURSES (1962–77)

Year	To maintain 1962 population/ personnel ratio	To improve over-all beds/ nurse ratio[a]	National- ization plan[b]	Payzin- Tekesin
1962	1,564	—	—	5,872
1964	1,676	3,784	76	6,227
1967	1,861	3,943	326	6,792
1972	2,218	5,554	724	7,859
1977	2,648	6,299	1,995	9,108

[a] Based on improved ratio of 20 beds/nurse, the standard set for nationalization plan hospitals.

[b] Based on the assumption that only $1/3$ of the nurses projected for nationalized areas will be in health centers while the other $2/3$ will be in hospitals.

TABLE 10–7. CUMULATIVE DEMAND PROJECTION FOR NURSES' AIDES (1962–77)

Year	To maintain 1962 population/ personnel ratio	To improve over-all beds/ nurse aide ratio[a]	Nationalization plan
1962	1,652	—	—
1964	1,762	5,045	53
1967	1,941	5,257	152
1972	2,285	7,769	336
1977	2,695	8,399	931

[a] Based on improved ratio of 15 beds/nurse aide.

16 percent* of all nurses will be required to staff training programs for nursing and midwifery personnel and MCH and health centers.

Nurses' Aides

Nurses' aides now almost equal the number of registered nurses. Under the nationalization plan only half as many nurses' aides are projected as compared to registered nurses (Table 10–7). Nurses' aides are to be used mainly for direct patient care in hospitals and therefore projected demand was based on a ratio of fifteen beds per nurses' aide.

*Based on the following low standards for teaching and supervision: 1 nurse per 10 students in higher nursing schools; 1 nurse per 20 students in health colleges, nursing schools, rural midwife schools, nurse's aide training courses; 1 nurse per MCH Center or health center.

Hospital Beds

Hospital care is expensive and requires proportionately a far greater investment of health personnel than other health activities. Although hospitals should receive relatively low priority in Turkey, certain minimum provisions are necessary as a base for other services. Even such minimum standards require a great increase in hospital beds (Table 10–8). The nationalization plan emphasizes ambulatory treatment through rural health units and as it extends westward, where most of the beds are now located, it will take over existing government hospitals. This explains the small number of new beds projected.

TABLE 10–8. CUMULATIVE PROJECTED DEMAND FOR HOSPITAL BEDS (1962–77)

Year	To maintain 1964 pop./bed ratio	New beds needed for nationalization plan[a]	Total demand for beds	Number of beds per 10,000 population
1962	69,588	—	69,588	—
1964	74,506	1,176	75,680	24.3
1967	82,234	6,628	78,862	23.2
1972	97,081	14,007	111,088	28.3
1977	114,813	11,166	125,979	27.7

[a] Based on scheduled progress of nationalization plan in both urban and rural areas. Bed/population standard used for nationalized areas was 10 beds/30,000 population. Estimates were calculated for each province separately and then totaled.

Projected Personnel Demand Comparing Ratios of Major Categories of Health Workers to Population

For comparison purposes a final table (Table 10–9) is included giving the personnel to population rates projected until 1977. The ratios were computed on the basis of total demand for each category of health personnel from previous calculations. Total demand for doctors included specialists and general practitioners required to maintain the 1962 personnel/population ratio plus the number required for the nationalization plan. Total demands for nurses and nurses' aides included the numbers required to improve the hospital bed/nurse ratio or the bed/nurses' aide ratio plus the numbers required for the nationalization plan. Total demands for midwives and for *saglik memurus* included the numbers required to maintain the 1962 personnel/population ratios together with the additional numbers required for the nationalization plan and the integrated plan for rural areas.

The dramatic demonstration of the relative imbalance of doctors to all other health personnel is clearly evident. Demand for doctors continues to exceed every other personnel category. The over-all rate of improvement in other categories of personnel is indicated by the column in Table 10–9 giving the ratio of other trained health personnel to doctors. The ratio rises gradually from 1.1/1 to 1.8/1 over a period of fifteen years, whereas a reasonable ratio in most countries is considered to be 10/1.

TABLE 10–9. PROJECTED PERSONNEL DEMAND RELATED TO POPULATION (1962–77) (PERSONNEL PER 100,000 POPULATION)

Year	Doctors	Nurses	Nurses' aides	Mid-wives	*Saglik memurus*	Ratios of all other trained health personnel to doctors
1962	32	5	6	22	12	1.1/M.D.
1964	34	12	16	14	12	1.6/M.D.
1967	37	13	16	18	14	1.6/M.D.
1972	42	16	21	36	19	2.2/M.D.
1977	54	18	20	39	20	1.8/M.D.

11

SUMMARY FINDINGS AND SYNTHESIS OF PROJECTIONS

Health manpower planning cannot remain the scholarly interest of a few research workers. It also should not become merely a casual and incidental activity of personnel bureaus in health services. This critical component of the development process requires intensive and serious research, new methodology, and accurate data. The long-range issues are too important to be based on the fragmentary information and impressionistic, though often realistic, appraisals that normally provide the basis for most administrative decisions.

This national "Health Manpower Study in Turkey" has been long-term and intensive. In this summary chapter, we will describe first the methodological advances that have been made in several new areas. A priority listing of manpower requirements in Turkey will then be presented. Each of these priority items will be discussed and relevant data obtained in this study will be summarized. Supply and demand projections will be synthesized. Cost analyses will then be related to an estimate of probable available resources.

METHODOLOGICAL ADVANCES

1. The advantage of studying the whole health manpower situation concurrently has been clearly shown. Turkey was found to have a health manpower hourglass instead of a pyramid. There is a large bulge of doctors on top, few trained paramedical and auxiliary workers in the middle, and a large mass of indigenous health workers at the bottom.

2. Clearer categorization of the names, status, and relationships of health personnel has resulted from the over-all analysis of health services (Table 11–1).

3. The trial of multiple alternative methodological approaches in obtaining an accurate census of physicians permitted direct evaluation of each. An incidental benefit for Turkey was a major revision of the system of registration and regular reporting of health personnel.

4. The professional problems which make the Turkish doctor today restless and dissatisfied were defined by using a detailed questionnaire with a 97 percent response rate in a 10 percent random sample of all doctors.

5. An evaluation was done of the pilot program in Mus Province, of the Turkish government's new plan for national health services. Although the study demonstrated the need for some administrative changes, it was clear that, in general, the program represents a tremendous advance in health care, especially for rural areas.

6. The confused inter-relationships between private and public sectors in medical care were studied through special surveys of private practitioners. Conditions of practice were defined and estimates of probable income made.

7. Special problems of rural medical service were studied in three groups of rural practitioners and a control group. A battery of tests to measure skills and attitudes relevant to rural service was adapted from a Johns Hopkins project in India.

8. In medical education, Turkey faces a crisis more acute than in most countries. Medical schools co-operated well in providing data about their problems. Clearer definition of the new orientation desired for doctors has permitted analysis of changes required in the teaching program.

9. Measurement of the supply of nurses was done by conducting a census. Specific problems were explored in a detailed questionnaire completed by 85 percent of a 30 percent sample. From this data career profiles of Turkish nurses were developed and the reasons for nursing shortages evaluated. Most other problems derive from the poor status of the profession and the negative attitudes of both doctors and the public.

10. Existing sources of information were used to estimate the supply of other health categories. Personnel for environmental sanitation are not clearly defined and almost nonexistent. The present *saglik memuru* is much too multipurpose to function efficiently.

TABLE 11–1. CATEGORIES AND EDUCATIONAL LEVELS OF HEALTH WORKERS IN TURKEY BY FUNCTIONAL GROUPS

	Medical care	General public health and communicable disease control	Nursing and midwifery	Sanitation	Technical and laboratory activities	Other paramedical functions
University-level and professional	Doctors and specialists	Public health doctors and Gevher Nesibe graduates	University-level nurses	Sanitary engineers (almost none available) civil engineers	Academic disciplines in basic laboratory sciences	Dentists, pharmacists
Middle level-lycee equivalents	Some *saglik memurus*	Public health nurses and some *saglik memurus*	Registered nurses and midwives	Some *saglik memurus*	Some *saglik memurus*	Some *saglik memurus*
Auxiliary level-trained personnel		Special assistants in malaria, trachoma, TB programs, etc.	Nurses' aides, rural midwives	Some rural *saglik memurus*		Some rural *saglik memurus*
Untrained and indigenous personnel	Needlemen, indigenous practitioners		Hastabakici			

11. Special data were collected on many indigenous health workers through the co-operation of social scientists conducting two village surveys. Numerically dominating the health scene is the ubiquitous "needleman," often an army medical corpsman who has returned to his home village, and the *ebe anne* or traditional birth attendant.

12. A survey was done of all health institutions. Data were obtained on personnel distribution and organizational arrangements. Particularly difficult methodologically, and therefore limited to only a few representative institutions, was an effort to analyze relative costs of various service functions.

13. Projection of supply was done using specified alternative assumptions.

14. Major methodological advances have been made in learning how to measure and project demand for health personnel. Planning based on biological need (scientifically determined burden of disease) or popular desire (health services people want) was discarded as having little immediate relevance to planning although these may become useful concepts later, when present shortages and discrepancies are reduced. Instead, estimates were based largely on technically and administratively feasible demand (feasible control measures with appropriate administrative framework to apply them) and on economic demand (activities for which society or individuals will and can pay). Present demand was quantified. Projected demand was based on specified assumptions and government plans.

PRIORITY LISTING OF MAJOR MANPOWER REQUIREMENTS

1. Nursing personnel:
   Over-all shortage.
   Lack of clear role definition and low prestige.
   Need for appropriate modification of educational programs.
2. Solution of professional problems of medical practitioners:
   Urban-rural distribution.
   Attitudes of doctors toward rural service.
   Overspecialization.
   Reduction of present unhappy mixture of private and salaried
      practice.
   Low productivity of doctors.
   Growing financial insecurity of doctors.
   Migration of doctors out of Turkey.

3. Family-planning personnel:
   No clear definition of relative contributions of various professionals and auxiliaries.
   Uncertain role of midwives.
   Responsibility for motivational activities not clearly specified.
4. Auxiliaries for rural medical care:
   Mass need in regionalized program of nationalized health services.
   Need for substituting trained and supervised personnel for 30,000 needlemen now practicing privately.
   Possible joint training program with Army for medical corpsmen.
5. Sanitation personnel:
   No clear personnel categories at either professional or auxiliary levels.
   Confused role of *saglik memuru*.
6. Medical education:
   Immediate prospects for increase in supply depend mainly on reducing dropouts and repeaters.
   Continuing need for reorientation of educational program to meet needs of modern Turkey.
7. Professional problems of public health practitioners:
   Low prestige and poor working conditions.
   Medico-legal responsibilities.
8. Administrative reorganization of National Health Services with appropriate modifications of nationalization plan.

SUMMARY DATA ON MAJOR MANPOWER PRIORITIES

Nursing Personnel

The shortage in nursing personnel has long been recognized; as a result of this study it has now been quantitated. There is an overall ratio of one nurse per 17,000 people, whereas for doctors the ratio is about one per 3,000 people. In other words, there are more than five doctors for every nurse in Turkey. Even more than doctors and hospitals, nurses tend to be concentrated in urban areas so that in southeastern Anatolia the ratio is one nurse for more than 94,000 people. Nurses give almost no direct care to patients in hospitals. Even trained nurses' aides are so few that when the number of nurses and nurses' aides are added, there are still two doctors to one individual with any kind of nurse training.

Since it has been generally accepted that family planning should be part of the regular health services in Turkey, most family-planning functions will be performed by regular health personnel, particularly in the nationalized health services. Women doctors will be most needed in parts of the country where conservatism causes women to prefer care from members of their own sex. We have little basis for judgment about the extent to which midwives with special training can be used. Their access to women during the antenatal and post-partum periods permits the building of confidence and rapport at times when the potential of family-planning acceptance seems to be maximal. Much remains to be done in studying the motivational process in family planning and the optimum personnel and approaches to be used in Turkey.

Auxiliaries for Mass Rural Medical Care

The most numerous health workers in Turkey are the needlemen and the indigenous practitioners who practice privately outside the regular health care system. They represent the big bottom bulge of the manpower hourglass. At least 30,000 needlemen inject penicillin and other chemotherapeutic agents promiscuously. Their only certification is their use of a syringe. Their limited training was acquired as an army medical corpsman or while working as a janitor or menial employee in a hospital. Together with indigenous untrained "birth attendants" and the many indigenous practitioners specializing in diverse therapeutic procedures such as pouring lead and writing spiritual charms, they constitute a major occupational group in whom the public has confidence and makes a sizable but unquantifiable financial investment.

Little can be done about bringing most untrained practitioners into the organized health services. On the other hand, it is becoming increasingly apparent that the rural health services will be more effective if new categories of medical care auxiliaries are developed. The new functions might include: preliminary screening and care of patients having common and minor illnesses, administration of the routine and simple therapeutic measures under the supervision of a doctor, and health education. Under medical supervision in a regionalized framework such individuals can also effectively staff subcenters in co-operation with basically trained rural midwives. At present, this medical assistant function is sometimes filled by *saglik memurus* who specialize in medical care without adequate preparation.

A possibility that deserves serious consideration is to develop a joint program with the Army so that medical corpsmen can be trained specifically for eventual employment in rural health services. The Ministry of Health would, of course, want to organize special training programs to orient these rural workers to their functions in the nationalized health services.

Personnel for Sanitation Services

As with family-planning personnel, little has been said in this study about sanitation personnel because there are essentially none of them to be studied. The three Turkish sanitary engineers we identified were trained in foreign schools and have worked either outside of the country or outside of sanitary engineering. Government agencies responsible for civil works do not have specialists in sanitary engineering since the planning and development of water and sewage facilities are considered part of general engineering. The recent appointment of a sanitary engineer to the Middle East Technical University faculty may bring some recognition of the relevance of this discipline to the health needs of Turkey.

It has been assumed that *saglik memurus* would fulfill sanitation functions in routine health services. They receive only cursory and superficial educational preparation in this field and are, therefore, essentially unprepared for work requiring much technical competence. In rural areas, however, *saglik memurus* have functioned effectively as general purpose health workers carrying out the relatively simple sanitary measures needed in a village community.

Specialization in sanitation is most needed at the middle manpower level. A beginning has been made by permitting *saglik memurus* to specialize in sanitation courses in health colleges. As an alternative, consideration should be given to setting up completely new training programs and career opportunities for sanitarians. As the water and sewage programs of urban areas expand, such individuals are needed immediately. Then as environmental health problems of modern urban life increase, especially food sanitation and air pollution, the demand for such persons will grow.

The Crisis in Medical Education

The tone of the total health services depends on the quality of medical education. In Turkey qualitative considerations are now more important than quantitative expansion. Because of the great financial investment in medical education, particular care must be taken in ensuring efficiency in operation of the medical schools.

The findings of this study suggest that the opening of new medical schools should be postponed. More can be gained at this stage by concentrating on improving the utilization and output of existing schools. Greater efficiency could be achieved by splitting the present Istanbul medical school into two schools. The enrollment of the remaining four medical schools could be expanded. The most obvious and quickly available quantitative expansion can be achieved by reducing dropouts and repeaters in the medical schools. Only 56 percent of all students admitted to medical schools actually graduate, yielding a dropout rate of 44 percent. A tremendous educational investment could be salvaged by improving selection practices and providing learning and examination conditions which would encourage medical students to carry through to graduation. It is apparent that the poor selection leads the faculty to use the high failure rate as a screening process. Thirty-two percent of admissions or 58 percent of graduated students required more than the specified six years of the medical curriculum to graduate. Many students put in extra years to compensate for inadequate preparation. It is unfortunate that some medical educators consider a high failure rate to be a status symbol and equate it with high academic standards.

The extra investment in repeaters and dropouts has been calculated to require the educational equivalent of two additional medical schools each graduating approximately 100 students a year. From our calculations of the cost of medical education this represents a loss of from 20–30,000,000 TL in capital expenses and at least 40,000,000 TL per year in operating expenses.

Ultimately more important are the long-range qualitative changes which must be made in medical education. The pattern of education is derived directly from the didactic teaching of German medical schools of the past century. The needs of Turkey today require a drastic revision of curriculum and teaching methods which can be achieved only with a new orientation in faculty members. More practical experience and direct involvement in problem solving would create confidence and competence in graduates. Specific emphases which were found to be deficient are: practical experience in the basic sciences; community-oriented basic courses such as social science, biostatistics, and epidemiology; practical clinical skills concentrating on the whole patient and his family environment; sound experience with common diseases of Turkey, especially infections and nutritional deficiencies; practical rural experience in the comprehensive clinical and preventive activities required of health center doctors; a new orientation in professional values appropriate to modern medicine in Turkey.

Professional Problems of Public Health Practitioners

Although public health and preventive medicine typically have maximum impact on a nation's health, these specialties are, in almost all countries, accorded the lowest prestige of the medical disciplines. In Turkey most public health positions have been filled by part-time doctors who give their major attention to private practice. Ministry of Health regulations list 103 duties to be performed by Medical Officers of Health, although very few of these doctors have had any special public health training. In the 10 percent sample survey, one-third of the doctors indicated that they had worked as an M.O.H. at some time. When asked about the problems of such service, one-third of the group indicated that the greatest problem was taking care of medicolegal cases; another one-third objected to the unsatisfactory working conditions with too much being expected for too little pay. Another common complaint was that the health officer is responsible to the *kaymakam* or head of the district government who often exercises undue control over technical aspects of the doctor's work. If public health and curative functions can be combined in a comprehensive health service such as the nationalization plan, many of the present difficulties should be resolved.

Administrative and Institutional Reorganization

Although long-range manpower planning obviously depends primarily on educational output, short-range targets such as those of the usual five-year plan can be met only by retraining or improving utilization of health personnel already available. Effective and efficient utilization of precious manpower resources depends largely on the administrative framework. A comprehensive analysis of the total institutional structure of Turkish health services showed clearly that investment in hospitals has been too great relative to other activities. Mass problems have been largely ignored. Investment in preventive services and ambulatory care has been distinctly secondary to the expensive inpatient care.

A major advance in health planning for Turkey was the Nationalization of Health Services Plan. In 1964, a Turkish member of our team evaluated the pilot project in Mus Province after it had been in operation a year. At the relatively small per capita annual

cost of 32 TL ($3.55) a dramatic expansion of health services oc-
curred. Clinical care was provided to 122,000 people in the pilot
year as compared to 13,000 in the previous year. The greatest increase was in ambulatory care in health units and in home care.
Auxiliary health personnel increased from 35 to 123 and most of
their effort went into preventive activities and health education.
An estimated 56 percent of the total annual health expenditure of
the province was devoted to prevention. National plans for specific
disease control programs such as malaria eradication and the new
National Family-Planning Program are to be integrated into this
regionalized structure. The integrated health services are an interim
plan to provide for the surveillance phase of malaria eradication.

SYNTHESIS OF SUPPLY AND DEMAND PROJECTIONS

The real pay-off in manpower studies comes when comparison
of supply and demand projections reveals shortages and discrepancies. Projected estimates of unmet demand are especially critical
for long-range educational planning since they provide the quantitative base for establishing priorities in educational expansion.

Doctors

In the present synthesis (Table 11–2), projected estimates of
supply and demand for physicians were compared. In this calculation, the various measures for improving medical school output
were combined to get maximum projected supply (Chapter 8).
Similarly, the conditions that would increase demand were combined to get total projected demand (Chapter 10). These projections include increases to match population growth plus the calculated new requirements of the nationalized and integrated plans.

The estimated projected demand in 1964 was 504 which is 1,027
less than the actual unmet demand in that year calculated (Chapter
9) from unfilled budgeted positions and urgently needed expansion.
The difference is not unexpected since the projections do not allow
for the problem of unfilled positions.

The most noteworthy finding from the synthesis of data is that
although the divergence between supply and demand projections
is not serious up to 1972, a sharp increase in unmet demand is
projected by 1977. The more than 1,000 doctors needed per year
are probably a mathematical artifact. The large increase in demand
is largely due to expansion of the nationalization plan to cover the
heavily populated western parts of the country. It is hoped that as

TABLE 11-2. SYNTHESIS OF SUPPLY AND DEMAND PROJECTIONS FOR DOCTORS (1964)

Year	Maximum supply projection	Present unmet demand	Total projected demand	Projected unmet demand	Projected demand for specialists	Projected demand for general practitioners
1964	10,000	1,531	10,504	504	7,406	3,098
1967	11,200	—	12,668	1,468	8,748	3,920
1972	14,200	—	16,482	2,282	11,041	5,441
1977	17,700[a]	—	24,401	6,701	15,696	8,705

[a] This includes regular annual increment plus increased graduates from two new medical schools and reduced dropouts and repeaters.

metropolitan and urban areas are included in full national coverage, existing government institutions and personnel will be included in the plan. The need for new doctors should not be as great as indicated in the calculations. In order to recruit doctors already in practice, the salary and service conditions will have to be favorable but recruitment should be easier than in eastern Anatolia since doctors will be able to stay in or near the more desirable urban areas.

Other data presented in this report suggest that unmet demand for medical services can be met best by improving utilization, distribution, and productivity of doctors. The present productivity of doctors, especially those in private practice, is extremely low. If more patients could afford their fees, doctors presumably would welcome them. Evaluation of the Mus Pilot Project showed a remarkable increase in productivity under nationalization, from 1,430 to 3,578 patients per year per doctor.

The demand projections also provide a basis for judging the balance of general practitioners and specialists required. By 1977, the number of specialists should be more than doubled, whereas the number of general practitioners should be more than tripled. This shift in balance will require deliberate efforts to moderate the present trend toward specialization.

Dentists and Pharmacists

The projections of demand for dentists and pharmacists were concentrated mainly on the limited requirements of the new nationalized health plan. Because of the adequate numbers projected at present rates of increase, it is probable that there will be plenty of these professionals for government services. Since they work almost entirely in the private sector, however, the apparent excess production can be readily absorbed in private practice. In fact, to fill the new positions being created the public sector will have to provide sufficient financial and other benefits to compete with the private sector.

Nurses

The shortage of nurses is greater than any of our summary calculations show. To maintain some semblance of achievable realism the standards for nurse demand have been set low. The total projected demand (Table 11–3) was obtained by adding the nurses needed in the nationalization plan to the nurses required to increase the ratio of nurses to hospital beds to 1/20 in each province. This is the standard set for the nationalization plan hospitals and is low by international standards. It does, however, give a somewhat inflated demand figure now because it will take time to reach these standards. In other words, the 1964 demand figure in this table has less significance than the targets in 1977. Similarly, the maximum supply projection is based on improved utilization of nursing schools which will require major changes in policy and educational practice. With such changes a tenfold decrease in the unmet demand by 1977 is possible. Finally, these projections will have meaning only if positions are created in the health services which provide nurses satisfying work opportunities and remuneration.

TABLE 11–3. SYNTHESIS OF SUPPLY AND DEMAND PROJECTIONS FOR NURSES (1964–77)

Year	Projected maximum supply[a]	Present unmet demand[b]	Projected total demand[c]	Projected unmet demand
1964	1,852	463	3,860	2,008
1967	2,696	—	4,269	1,573
1972	5,040	—	6,278	1,283
1977	8,008	—	8,294	286

[a] Based on maximum utilization of existing schools and a 62.5 annual activity rate of all graduate nurses.

[b] Under-reported. This includes only the unfilled budgeted positions reported by the Ministry of Health in 1964.

[c] Includes projected demand for nurses required to improve the bed/nurse ratio to 20 beds/nurse. This provides 15 percent of all nurses for training programs and health centers. 1964 projection provides for an average of 3 R.N.'s per hospital, 1 nurse-teacher per 20 students in training programs at lycee and middle-school levels, 1 nurse-teacher per 10 students at university level, 1 nurse per MCH or Health Center for OPD and home care.

Nurses' Aides

Nurses' aides are required in even greater numbers than nurses. The total demand projections require a great increase over present hospital staffing patterns (Table 11–4). The ratio of nurses' aides to hospital beds was projected to increase to 1/15. As with nurses, this gives a somewhat inflated figure for 1964 but provides a reasonable target for 1977. If steps are taken to provide the maximum projected supply the unmet demand in 1977 should be reduced to one half the present deficiency.

TABLE 11–4. SYNTHESIS OF PROJECTED SUPPLY AND DEMAND FOR TURKISH NURSES'
AIDES (1964–77)

Year	Projected maximum supply	Present unmet demand[a]	Projected total demand[b]	Projected unmet demand
1964	2,206	474	5,098	2,892
1967	3,210	—	5,409	2,199
1972	5,538	—	8,105	2,567
1977	7,865	—	9,330	1,465

[a] Under-reported. Includes only Ministry of Health report of unfilled budgeted positions.

[b] Based on improved ratio of 15 beds/nurse's aide.

Saglik Memurus

Projections were made of the supply and demand for *saglik memurus* even though the role of this category of health worker must be drastically revised and clarified. Under present circumstances there is only moderate projected demand. At the current rate of increment supply will exceed demand by approximately 2,000 for each five-year period (Table 11–5). If demand accelerates because of separation of the job responsibilities of *saglik memurus* into two or more subspecialties or even if new categories of health workers are developed, there should be no difficulty in recruiting young men into this type of work.

TABLE 11–5. SYNTHESIS OF SUPPLY AND DEMAND PROJECTIONS OF *Saglik Memurus* (1964–77)

Year	Maximum projected supply	Present unmet demand	Total projected demand	Excess production
1964	5,996[a]	343	3,798	2,198
1967	7,226[b]	—	4,631[c]	2,595
1972	9,276	—	7,458	1,818
1977	11,326	—	9,328	1,998

[a] Ministry of Health figures for end of 1964.

[b] Based on 409 (rounded off to 410) graduates per year. Increased output beyond that figure will probably compensate for attrition which was not calculated.

[c] Number needed for new Ministry of Health positions.

Midwives

No category of health personnel will be demanded in greater numbers in the new nationalized health services than rural midwives (Table 11–6). Many midwives are now working in the private sector, especially in the cities. Only 52 percent are in government services. Because they are not included in the national plans, urban midwives were not included in the projections. In addition, the new national family-planning program will use this category of personnel extensively. By 1977, the projected unmet demand will be 8,118. Such a massive increase in health manpower can be achieved only through an even more intensive and focused effort than is now intended.

TABLE 11–6. SYNTHESIS OF SUPPLY AND DEMAND PROJECTIONS OF RURAL[a]
MIDWIVES (1964–77)

Year	Maximum supply projections	Present unmet demand	Total projected demand	Projected unmet demand
1964	3,104[b]	679[d]	4,400	1,296
1967	4,604[c]	—	6,252	1,648
1972	7,104	—	14,148	7,044
1977	9,604	—	17,722	8,118

[a] Urban midwives are not included because they are not included in the nationalization and integration plans.

[b] Ministry of Health figures for end of 1964.

[c] About 500 graduates per year expected as village midwifery schools accelerate, estimated excess of output over attrition.

[d] Number still needed to fill Ministry of Health positions in 1964.

The government has already planned to considerably increase the number and distribution of health schools where rural midwives are trained. Even though a threefold increase in supply is projected, this is only one half the projected demand. More health schools must be opened, even though the greatest weakness in this program at present is that existing health schools are inadequately staffed. The first concentrated effort then must be to prepare sufficient numbers of midwives to work as full-time teachers in these schools. A particular problem is that these schools should be widely distributed in rural areas where it is difficult to get qualified teachers to go. Considerable innovative thinking will be required to meet this major challenge.

12

RECOMMENDATIONS

After the data collection and analysis phases of this health man-power study were completed, it seemed desirable to turn for interpretations and recommendations to the officials directly responsible for health policy and operations in Turkey. Their recommendations would have the great advantage of being feasible and practical. The fact that responsible Turkish decision-makers had been involved personally in working out the recommendations would increase the prospect of direct implementation.

The first step was to hold a conference on interpretation of the health manpower findings at the School of Public Health in Ankara in June, 1966. With the official impetus of the presence of three ministers, many representatives from the Ministry of Health, the Ministry of Education, the State Planning Organization, various directorates of the government, universities, professional schools, and all categories of health workers met for three days of intensive discussion and critical analysis. A draft of the report had been translated into Turkish and circulated. Data were evaluated and suggestions made for improving their validity. Preliminary recommendations were developed. One result of the discussion was that considerable redrafting of the manuscript proved necessary and two chapters were largely rewritten. With the additional data that were gathered and the revised interpretations, the text was approved by Turkish health authorities for publication.

The Ministry of Health then held a conference on implementation of the health manpower findings in December, 1966. This was a smaller meeting composed mainly of the heads of the various directorates of the health ministry. Most officials responsible for specific health programs were present. Again in three days of discussion, effort was focused to produce a set of recommendations which would have a reasonable chance of being implemented. The statement which follows is a redrafting of the recommendations from the conference. Prior to this conference and also subsequent to it, committees of the Ministry of Health and the Ankara School of Public Health put an impressive amount of time and effort into reviewing the research findings, evaluating their validity, and making drafts of the recommendations. Although there is some overlapping with the summary in the previous chapter, these recommendations are presented because of the important consideration that they were generated by and agreed to by the policy-makers and administrators of the health services of Turkey.

STATEMENT OF HEALTH PRIORITIES

Review of the health status of Turkey suggests that the following conditions should receive priority attention:

1. Among health problems, control of the following needs emphasis: infectious diseases (especially gastrointestinal and respiratory), malnutrition, sanitation, and maternal and child health. An immediate and urgent health problem is the rapid rate of population increase.

2. In data-gathering, considerably more attention must be given to basic epidemiological investigations of the incidence, prevalence, and distribution of disease; to improved registration of vital data such as deaths, births, population distribution and movement; and to the recording of information on environmental factors influencing health. Responsibility for each of these functions must be shared by the assigned government agencies and appropriate institutions.

3. In the organization of health services, far more attention should be given to preventive medicine and public health than to the curative services which have received more than their appropriate share of financial and personnel resources. Similarly, within the curative services the balance should be shifted away from hospital inpatient services to ambulatory care centers and services.

ADMINISTRATIVE CHANGES RELATING TO MANPOWER POLICY

Professional Registration and Periodic Censuses

Although most professionals are supposed to register to get a license to practice, no continuing system of reporting provides information about the activity, distribution, continuing education, and working status of health personnel. The registration office in the Ministry of Health should be strengthened and the new system of maintaining up-to-date files on all personnel as developed in this research should be made a continuing routine. All professionals should be required to report pertinent data about themselves at regular intervals. Co-operative relations with professional associations and pharmaceutical companies will help in maintaining these records.

Improved Utilization and Productivity of Health Personnel

Poor utilization and inadequate productivity of health manpower are the greatest deterrents to effective health services in Turkey today. Doctors see far too few patients in a day's work and much of their time is spent in performing tasks that could be done more efficiently and perhaps more effectively by properly trained middle-level and ancillary personnel. This includes particularly the inefficient system in hospitals of doctors personally supervising the nursing care provided by untrained *hastabakicis*. The greatest need in planning Turkey's health services is for studies of the manpower mix so that the special talents and training of each category of personnel will be used for tasks which can be done most efficiently by them with routine tasks being delegated down to the lowest possible manpower level.

Distribution of Personnel

Gross inequities now exist in the health services available to various segments of the Turkish population. The greatest need for equalization is in rural-urban distribution but closely related are the geographical distribution problems of eastern Turkey. This situation must improve rapidly because of political and economic pressures as well as the obvious humanitarian reasons.

Reorganization of Health Services in the Nationalization Plan

Many of the over-all health manpower deficiencies can be corrected in the progressive improvement and expansion of the nationalized health services. This program must, however, be adequately implemented and consolidated in each province where it is started before too rapid expansion is undertaken. To increase productivity, it is important to strengthen morale by providing a more consistent administrative framework, better working and living conditions, and appropriate economic incentives.

Future Health Manpower Planning within the Health Ministry and the School of Public Health in Ankara

To follow up this study a unit should be developed which will be responsible for the continued development of health manpower planning. This should be jointly staffed by the School of Public Health and the Ministry of Health. Planning is a continuing process which improves progressively through feedback from efforts at implementation.

MODIFICATIONS IN WORKING ARRANGEMENTS AND SERVICE CONDITIONS TO IMPROVE THE PRODUCTIVITY OF VARIOUS CATEGORIES OF HEALTH PERSONNEL

Doctors

The following specific recommendations are designed to improve the effectiveness and productivity of doctors.

a. Financial incentives and stability must be provided to remove the present financial insecurity which leads doctors to: work at two, three, or four jobs, migrate from the country, concentrate in cities, and overspecialize.

b. The tendency toward specialization must be moderated because the greater need is for general practitioners. One solution is to increase the prestige and pay of the general practitioner. Another is to establish far more stringent controls of the indiscriminate and poorly organized specialist training programs in hospitals.

c. Private practice—The proportion of doctors in full-time private practice will probably increase gradually as general economic conditions in Turkey improve. At present, the combination of public service with part-time private practice has deleterious effects on both systems. Doctors in public service should be encouraged both financially and professionally to limit their work to the basic job for which they are hired.

d. Standardization of government services—Turkey has at least five different systems of government medicine with different conditions of service and pay scales. The confusion can be alleviated only by some standardization.

e. Rural services—The tremendous needs of rural areas demand some equalization of the distribution of doctors. To permit villagers at least minimal access to medical care, the doctor can extend his range of services through trained intermediaries on the health team. To improve the quality of service of doctors working in rural areas the following immediately practical recommendations are made: a flexible wage scale should provide special allowances for remote and difficult areas; improved and increased amounts of medical supplies and equipment must be regularly available; supervisory control in a regional framework should be by doctors experienced in rural health and community problems rather than by non-medical or inexperienced individuals; sufficient numbers of adequately trained paramedical and auxiliary personnel must be available; educational facilities should be provided for children of health personnel working in rural areas; a workable rotation system should be established to allow doctors to be moved on to more desirable locations and educational opportunities after a period of service under difficult conditions; supervisory relationships within the administrative hierarchy should be a part of in-service training rather than just inspection.

f. Responsibility for medicolegal services—Government doctors now have to spend a disproportionate amount of their time on medicolegal problems. Many of these could be handled by other government officials, thus relieving the doctors for medical and other professional duties.

g. Community medicine specialization—The nationalization plan will require a new community orientation in doctors. To ensure this emphasis in the service generally there must be a rapid increase in specialists in community medicine and public health. If such a specialty is given adequate status to attract good people, it will improve community care by all physicians.

h. Compulsory service for doctors—Since university education in Turkey is essentially free there is considerable logic behind the requirement that all medical graduates serve a specified period of time in a situation assigned at the discretion of the Ministry of Health. If such a decision is made, particular care must be taken to avoid favoritism in appointments because this will undermine the morale of the whole service.

Dentists and Pharmacists

A more balanced distribution of dentists and pharmacists should be encouraged. At present most are in private practice and concentrated in metropolitan centers. Under the nationalization plan, a small proportion of dentists and pharmacists will be employed at regional medical centers. Auxiliary personnel in these fields should be provided.

Nurses and Nurses' Aides

Nursing should be recognized as a separate profession. Considerable independence should be given to nurses in developing their distinctive contributions to health care.

a. Clear differentiation must be made between the three levels of nurses. Uniforms of various types and colors should be worn to assist the public and hospital personnel in recognizing each category. It is recommended that specification of these distinctions be carried out in a special conference or working group authorized by the government to review and revise the organization of nursing services.

(1) A new title signifying their professional status should be found for university graduates in nursing. They must be accorded the prestige, position, supervisory and educational status, responsibilities, and perquisites appropriate to such professional status.

(2) Registered nurses who are graduates of health colleges at the lycee level should also be given an appropriate title. Their responsibilities, role and status should be clearly defined together with appropriate compensations and living conditions.

(3) Large numbers of nurses' aides must be graduated from health schools. Again their role and status need to be clearly defined. This group probably can most appropriately use the traditional title *hemsire*.

(4) For male students who are accepted in the nursing sections of health colleges, a suitable title should be found which has no feminine connotation. Again a clear definition of role and responsibilities must be made.

b. The working hours of all categories of personnel providing nursing services must be revised. At present the excessive hours on duty interfere with efficient service and recruitment.

c. A large pool of experienced and mature nurses is available among the married graduates whose children are away in school. Major adjustments in working conditions should include modifying the working hours to times suitable for women with family responsibilities and providing a living allowance to compensate for the room and board received by other nurses.

d. Because one-third of the nurses in the nationalized health services will work in ambulatory services, primarily as public health nurses, particular attention should be given to preparing them for community and preventive responsibilities.

Midwives

a. Although midwives can be quickly trained and probably easily recruited, it will require careful logistic and educational planning to meet the tremendous demand. The rural midwife can work efficiently only if she has adequate supervision and a new working relationship must be developed reaching out from rural health centers to maintain continuing contact with the midwives who will be stationed in isolated and remote situations.

b. Specific role responsibilities and effective working methods have not been developed yet in family planning, but it is particularly important that field investigations be done to find out how rural midwives can contribute best to this new activity.

Saglik Memurus

a. The *saglik memuru* is now in an anomalous and ambiguous position. He is expected to do almost everything and yet is prepared to do very little. The six different types of responsibility (medical care assistant, sanitation, laboratory and x-ray technician, statistical clerk, and pharmacist) now imposed on them should be clearly distinguished. He should be able to concentrate in only one area both in preparation and work. Within that area of concentration, he should then be able to improve his competence and advance in the administrative services.

b. *Saglik memurus* tend to be distributed geographically over the country more widely than almost any other category of health personnel. In the provinces, however, they are still concentrated in urban areas and the nationalization plan should ensure their distribution to the rural areas where they are most needed.

Sanitation Personnel

Almost nothing has been done about developing personnel to provide sanitation services. If sanitary engineers and lower level sanitation personnel are not developed, then selected *saglik memurus* should receive considerably more training and experience in this discipline.

Rural Medical Assistants

To increase the effective range of doctors' work in rural health centers and to improve their productivity in medical care, adequate numbers of medical assistants should be provided. One possibility is that a large number of male nurses or *saglik memurus* should be trained but they should probably be given a new name. A simpler alternative for a lower level rural auxiliary is to work out a new relationship with the Army so that individuals who are already being trained as medical corpsmen can be effectively used when they return to civilian life. Following their basic training in the Army they can be given further training under the Ministry of Health to be able to do preliminary diagnostic screening of patients as they come to health centers and subunits and to treat minor ailments while referring all patients with any indication of serious illness to the doctor. They should also be able to provide much of the continuing routine therapy of complicated cases under the direction of the doctor. Under supervision such health personnel should gradually take over much of the mass medical care responsibility of rural areas. The present vacuum has been filled by needlemen, indigenous practitioners, and untrained midwives.

MODIFICATIONS OF EDUCATIONAL PROGRAMS

Medical Education

a. The greatest immediate priority needs in medical education are qualitative rather than quantitative. By 1977, to provide a moderate increase in doctors the number and enrollment of medical schools should gradually expand as appropriate faculty and facilities can be provided.

b. Curriculum changes in the basic sciences should be directed mainly toward increasing their practical relevance to the everyday work of the physicians. Opportunities for practical clinical experience should include health conditions which are prevalent locally, especially the common infections and nutritional deficiencies. In order for doctors to take responsibility for whole communities in nationalized health services, they should be specifically prepared in the basis sciences of community medicine including the social sciences, statistics, and epidemiology.

c. Because the greatest need in Turkey today is for rural doctors, the educational program should provide for experience in rural areas; the teaching staff should include individuals who have had solid preparation and experience in rural work. Another major emphasis in medical education should be on the preventive and public health activities which are an increasing component of comprehensive health care.

Nursing Education

a. Following specific categorization and job definition at each of the various levels of nursing, the curriculum of nursing schools must be fitted to the particular responsibilities which nurses will fill.

b. The acute shortage of nursing faculty members makes it inadvisable to open more new schools at this time. The urgently needed quantitative increase in numbers of nurses can be achieved by improving the utilization of existing schools. Most schools have extremely small graduating classes and an increase to fifty graduates per year from schools which admit only women and twenty-five female nurses per year from coeducational schools is feasible if faculty and facilities are strengthened.

c. In medical schools and all other schools for health professionals opportunities to work with nurses and learn about nursing should be included. This would help other health personnel to develop an appropriate respect for nurses and their work.

Midwifery Education

In the massive expansion of health schools for rural midwives most attention needs to be paid to the provision of faculty since the few teachers now are only part time. Special inducements will be needed to attract qualified teachers to the rural areas.

SUMMARY GENERALIZATIONS

Two important generalizations in manpower planning grow out of these varied analyses. First, manpower availability can be increased more efficiently and rapidly by improving utilization of personnel already available and especially by making more appropriate use of existing educational institutions. Second, of the qualitative considerations in educational planning the most important relate to the development of the service values and attitudes which determine the ultimate productivity, effectiveness, and quality of all personnel and these depend mainly on the values and attitudes of their teachers and of their immediate supervisors in the health services.

INDEX

Administration: provincial and local 8, 11–12, 58; reorganization, 41, 52, 55, 105, 288–89; Ministry of Health, 59, 192–95, 197–200, 244–48; inefficient practices, 61; health center, 90, 198–99; medical schools, 107; nursing, 127, 130, 145, 151; budgeted positions, 128, 151, 230–31; medical officers of health, 192; provincial directorates, 192–94, 198–200; public health services, 244–48

Agency for International Development, ix, x

Ankara School of Public Health; viii, 13, 15, 114, 209, 288

Birth rates, 14, 174

Birth records, 10–11

Bone-setter, 179, 181, 183, 186, 188–90

Circumciser, 179, 183, 186, 189–90

Communicable disease control, 15–17, 19–25, 90, 247; malaria, 20–22, 192, 198, 200–1, 204; tuberculosis, 15–16, 193, 198, 204–5; budgetary provision, 209–10

Community medicine, teaching, 109, 113–15, 126; recommendations, 291. *See also* Preventive medicine; Public health

Curative medicine, vii, 198; patient load, 67–69; integration with preventive, 100–1; cost of health services, 206

Death rates: crude, 12, 14; infant, 13–14, 17, 175; tuberculosis, 15; measles, 20; malnutrition, 29

Dentists, 163–65, 213; education, 163–64; income, 164; distribution, 164–65; demand projections, 259, 263; recommendations, 291

Diseases, 11–32; tuberculosis, 13, 15–16; pneumonia, 13, 203; heart and vascular, 13; intestinal infections, 17–19, 203; communicable, 19–24; quarantinable, 24–25. *See also* Communicable disease control

Doctors: census, 33–40; professional problems, 40–63; income, 47–50, 73–81, 88; private practice, 63–81; attitudes toward rural service, 82–104;

medical education, 104–26; supply projections, 214–18; productivity, 232–33; demand projections, 261–63; synthesis of supply and demand, 281–83; recommendations for change, 290–91. *See also* General practitioners; Private practice; Specialists, clinical

Economy: growth, 2; educational expenditures, 4; demand for health services, 226–31

Education: general system, 2–9; preuniversity, 2–4; expenditures, 4; present demand for educational institutions and staff, 249–50; of health workers, 269–70. *See also* Medical education; Nursing education; Midwifery education

Family planning program, 14, 82, 189–91, 214, 276–77; midwives, 171, 175–76, 286; recommendations, 293, 295

Five-year plan, ix, 2, 119, 215

General practitioners, 37–38, 53–55, 88, 214, 275–76, 281–83; private practice, 66–67; income, 74–80; attitudes toward general practice, 86, 97; demand projections, 259, 262–63. *See also* Doctors; Private practice

Health center: doctors' attitudes toward rural service, 82–104; doctors' financial expectations, 88, 100; factors influencing recruitment, 100; bed capacity, 194–96, 240; administration, 194, 198–99; satellite stations, 198–99; staffing pattern, 198–99; fees for service, 199–200; staff salaries, 200; Mus pilot project, 201–6; curative health services, 206; budgetary provisions, 209–10; patient load, 232–33; cost, 236–39, 249

Health education, 201, 204, 281

Health technician, *See Saglik memuru*

Health workers: interrelationships, 182–89

Hospitals: general, 55, 193–98; residencies, 55; staffing pattern, 138–39, 145, 224, 243, 250–51; geographical distribution, 144–46, 240; bed capacity, 194–98, 240; teaching hospitals, 195;

THE JOHNS HOPKINS PRESS

Designed by Arlene J. Sheer

Composed in Monotype Baskerville by
Baltimore Type and Composition Corporation

Printed offset by Universal Lithographers, Inc.
on 60-lb P & S, R

Bound by L. H. Jenkins, Inc. in Columbia Riverside Linen